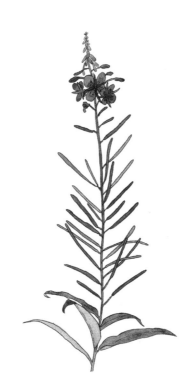

Quarto.com

© 2025 Quarto Publishing Group USA Inc.
Text © 2025 Lori Snyder

First Published in 2025 by Cool Springs Press, an imprint of The Quarto Group,
100 Cummings Center, Suite 265-D, Beverly, MA 01915, USA.
T (978) 282-9590 F (978) 283-2742

Cool Springs Press titles are also available at discount for retail, wholesale, promotional, and bulk purchase. For details, contact the Special Sales Manager by email at specialsales@quarto.com or by mail at The Quarto Group, Attn: Special Sales Manager, 100 Cummings Center, Suite 265-D, Beverly, MA 01915, USA.

29 28 27 26 25   1 2 3 4 5

ISBN: 978-0-7603-9325-3

Digital edition published in 2025
eISBN: 978-0-7603-9326-0

Library of Congress Control Number: 2024947532

Design and Page Layout: Justin Page
Photography: pages 5, 8–10, 13, 14, 17, 18, 20, 23, 24, 26, 218, 220, 224–226, 230, 234, 235 (right) by Belinda White at The Twining Trail; pages 149, 151, 167, 171, 215 by Alamy; page 235 (left) by Scott McAlpine; all others are Shutterstock
Illustration: Julia Alards-Tomalin

Printed in China

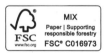

MIX
Paper | Supporting responsible forestry
FSC www.fsc.org FSC® C016973

Disclaimer
This is your journey, an important one for a good and healthy life. Whether you are new to herbal medicine or experienced, please start slowly and listen to your body. Food and plants can react differently in every body and can have an effect on other medicines and foods. Spend time with someone local who knows about plants to deepen your learning. Seek advice from a trusted health care provider before use. Above all else, take great responsibility for your health.

LoriAnn Bird

Indigenous Métis Herbalist

REVERED ROOTS

Ancestral teachings
and wisdom
of wild, edible,
and medicinal
plants

COOL
SPRINGS
PRESS

Deep Gratitude

I acknowledge that I reside on the unceded and stolen lands of the Coast Salish Peoples. Known colonially as Vancouver, the three Nations, the Original Inhabitants are: the xʷməθkwəy̓əm (Musqueam), Skwxwú7mesh (Squamish), and Səl̓ílwətaʔ/Selilwitulh (Tsleil-Waututh) Nations. It is my responsibility to state the "truth and reconcile," for us not to admit the genocide, the stolen children, the residential schools, and the missing and murdered people who have been lost to the imperial colonial system that now presides over these lands and waters. We must feel the discomfort, speak the truth of the history and make right relations, apologize and concile with our neighbors, so we can move forward with collaboration, co-creating a better future for our children's children. May we be good ancestors.

LoriAnn Bird

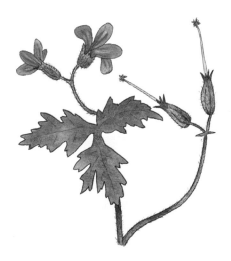

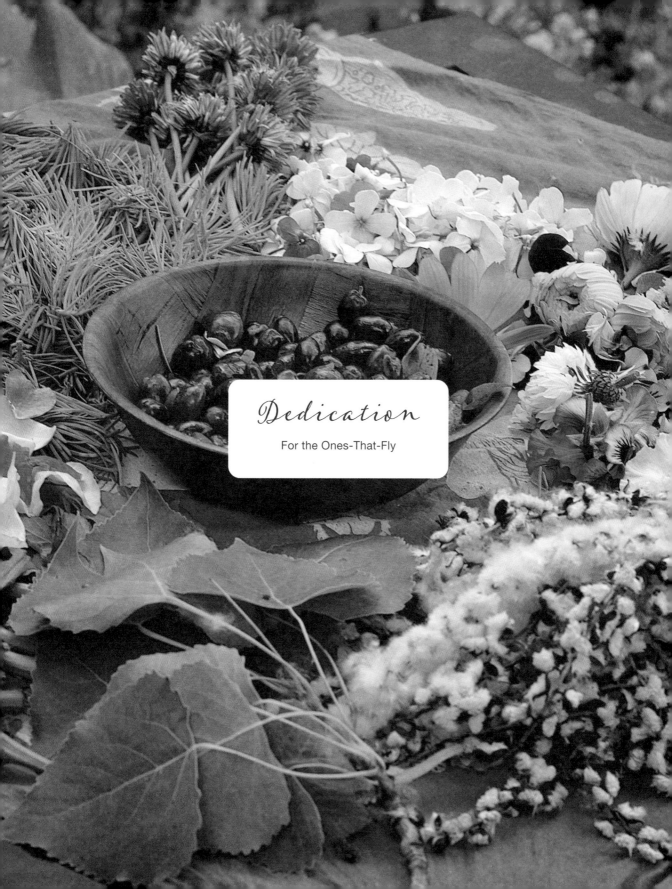

Dedication

For the Ones-That-Fly

Contents

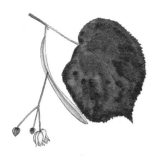

☷☷☷ AUTUMN: *Harvesting Before Hibernation*

☷☷☷ WINTER: *Slowing Down to Rest and Dream*

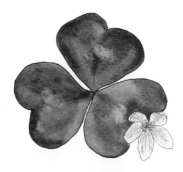

PART III

ALL OUR RELATIONS

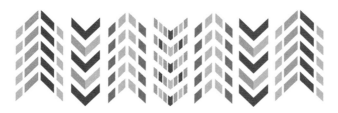

It's the beginning of a new year and the soft rain clouds have expanded from the heavens down, touching the Salish Sea on the West Coast of Turtle Island. The view of the North Shore Mountains, home of the "Two Sisters" Mountain, known as *Ch'ich'iyuy Elxwikn* by the Squamish People, is shrouded in mist. Like a blank canvas inviting us, you and me, to start again remembering our connection to Mother Earth and all that exists.

I live here, on what is now called Vancouver, Canada, on occupied territories of three Nations, xʷməθkwəy̓əm (Musqueam), Skwxwú7mesh (Squamish), and the Səl̓ílwəta?/Selilwitulh (Tsleil-Waututh). The people here have a deep understanding, agreements, protocols, instructions, and ways of being that have been shared for generations. I hold my hands up with deep gratitude and reverence for this place that has instilled in me a love for all life. These lands and waters have shared knowledge to guide us, as the "Two-Leggeds" (humans), to live in a good way, to enjoy long, healthy lives, appreciating the richness and abundance that flourished here at one time.

I am an Indigenous Métis woman, mother of two beautiful bright daughters, an herbalist, a storyteller, and an educator of wild, native, and medicinal plants. As a curious seeker who loves to share teachings, I humbly trust that this book replants the seeds of remembering who we are. We are known as the Two-Leggeds, the youngest child of our community living with all that exists here on Mother Earth. I invite you on this journey to reclaim ancestral knowledge, to pass it on to your family, and to walk again in beauty, in harmony with nature.

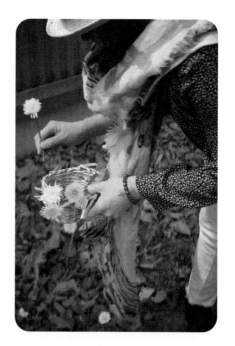

We can study and learn about plant medicines, but until we actually experience their gifts, they will always stay as knowledge or information. Our authority lies in our experience, which shapes and opens us. Information seldom changes minds. When we feel the grief and discomfort of our (humanity's) poor behavior in our hearts is when we change our minds. I trust the wisdom of plants

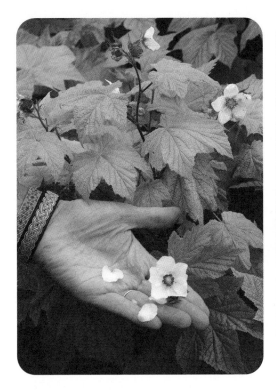
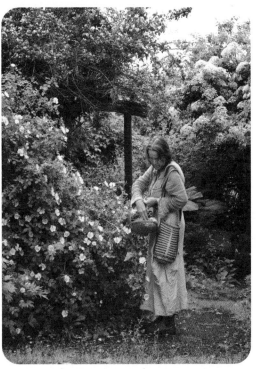

to heal, nourish, and guide us on how to live long, strong, healthy lives. To be in reciprocity and in right relationship with our More-Than-Human-Kin helps us understand our responsibility to our home and to express deep reverence for the gift of life. That's regenerative.

Once at a workshop, a woman shared how sorry she was that she had not taken notes when she walked with her grandmother. All the knowledge her grandmother held she would not be able to pass on to her grandchildren. Someone in the group said, "The plants remember." May this book reignite our traditions of passing on Earth's teachings, of learning about the wild weeds and the native plants that have long existed on Turtle Island, along with the medicine plants our ancestors brought over to Turtle Island from elsewhere. Seeds travel the wind, and so do we. Let's start by getting to know our plant teachers, the Rooted Nations. May this guide you back home.

The truth is, there could be a book dedicated to each plant. I want to offer you the beginnings. Which of these gifts speak to you? Go out and explore, seek, and question—with openness and inquiry. I have collected the teachings from my lifetime so far, but my education is far from over. I am now 61 and with grace and ease, I trust I will live to 104, to keep sharing the wisdom of wild, native, and medicinal plants.

This guidebook is created for you from the notes and research I have been collecting for a long time. May this book reignite our traditions of passing on knowledge. Earth teachings. As a messenger, this is the gift for you.

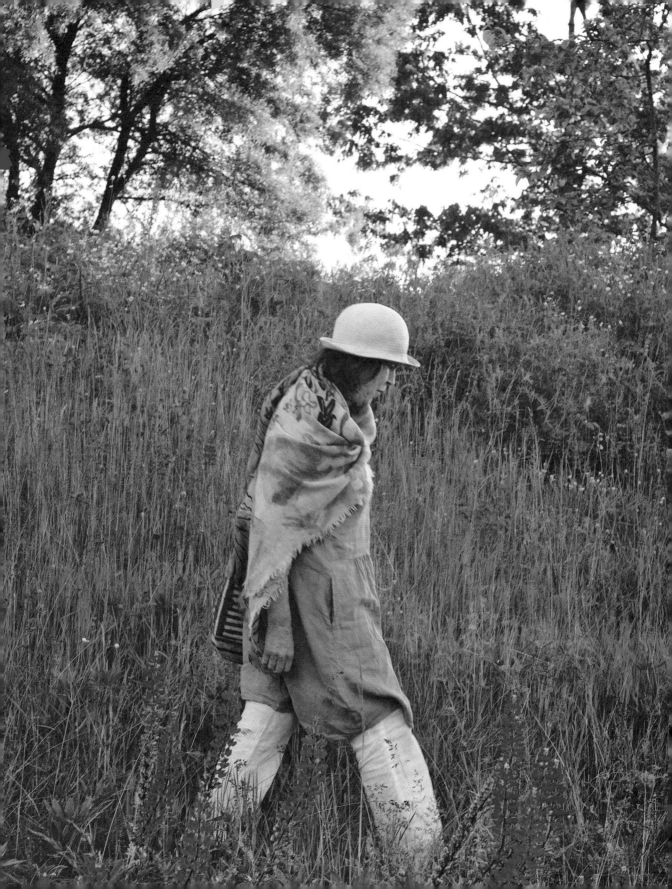

Reclaiming
Our History

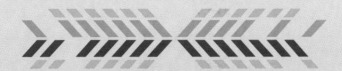

I have been reflecting on my ancestral history and the mandate of the Canadian government's policy to erase my cultural history. It is difficult to think about how much malice and fear the Canadian government had in the 1800s to behave this way, to remove the diversity of our planet's knowledge and the deep wisdom held in language, culture, stories, song, plants, animals, and rituals that emerged from the lands and waters of place. The celebration of the turning of the seasons, the constellations, and the movement of the moon is intrinsic to who we are.

Reclaiming our ancestral history is crucial at this time in history. I did not grow up knowing about my cultural heritage until, one day, I was asked about my ancestry. I was stunned by the question, and a flood of emotions, thoughts, and wonderment came to mind. I started to inquire and prayed for guidance to answer this question and to retrieve my relatives' past. I was led to an Indigenous healing circle, where I sat and listened, and when it was my opportunity to speak, I cried. I realized I did not know anything about my ancestral lineage. The journey is never-ending, as I have been letting go of the Euro-centric view I grew up with, along with confronting the political narrative of the past. It is frustrating to see the parallels today.

Mother Earth is known as *Pachamama* by the Incas and as *Aluna* by the Kogi People from Columbia. For the Aztecs, the Mother was called *Tonantzin*. The Hindu spoke of *Bhumi Devi*, the goddess of Earth. In the Greek language, Gaia. In China, the Earth goddess is *Hou Tu*.

In the Ojibwa language as shared by Larry Aitken from Leech Lake Tribal College, we can speak out loud the name of *ni-maamaa-aki*, the spirit who oversees the four principles: 1. soil (earth covering), 2. plants, 3. animals, and 4. people.

Reclaiming our roots activates the body's memory, the DNA, our family stories. Our native tongues contain teachings on how we "show good manners" and grasp the cosmology of our origins.

We are born with two physical parents and two spiritual parents according to the teachings of the Indigenous People of the Andes, the Q'ero People. Teachings come from many places on our magnificent planet, and we can give many names to this invisible energy, the source that guides us. I was not exposed to any of these teachings while I was growing up. Today, I am open to all teachings that speak to my heart. My experience brings to mind that knowledge comes from the land, waters, all our relations, and all that exists. I am deeply grateful for the guidance that helps keep me grounded in this wonderment of life from all the Elders, guides, and teachers—both seen and unseen—along the way.

Uncovering the history of my ancestors was daunting as my family spoke little about the past. I was guided to the place where the horizon expands on an endless landscape and arrived on the most recent homeland of my ancestors: the big open skies of the prairies. At the St. Boniface Historical Society, which specializes in Métis genealogy, I provided the names of my family and within a few weeks I received a booklet with names, dates, articles, and photocopies of deeds that tracked my lineage back to the 1600s, crossing the ocean from France. A clue connecting back to my Indigenous Grandmothers from the Cree Nations, the Tsuut'ina (Sarcee), who are part of the Dene, Athabaskan People, and the Anishinaabeg (plural) First Nations. The Anishinaabeg encompass groups of culturally and linguistically distinct peoples, like the Ojibwe, Saulteaux, and Nipissing. All are listed in the document. My ancestors are known as the Red River Métis People, a blend of Indigenous and European.

Reading *The North-West Is Our Mother* by Jean Teillet and *Gabriel Dumont* by George Woodcock revealed a passage of my lost past, including our way of life, our culture, and our language and protocols that supported sovereignty. Known as Sky Watchers or Wayfinders, we followed the movement of the stars, guiding seasonal hunting and celebrations. In the constellations of Ursa Major, within the Big Dipper, at the bottom of the bowl, are the pointer stars. They are pointing to Polaris, the unmoving North Star, a directional indicator. All the other constellations dance around Polaris. Not only guiding Indigenous cultures, stars like Polaris also guided enslaved peoples to find freedom in the North. The interweaving of Father Sky and Mother Earth grounds our cultural beliefs and practices, affirming our interconnectedness to all that exists. Our connection to the sky is found in cultures worldwide. I have a deep gratitude for all the knowledge keepers like Wilfred Buck, a Cree knowledge holder who shares these stories so that we can pass them down once again to the children.

Let us turn off the city lights twice a month during the new moon and full moon so we can reintroduce our children to the Milky Way and the constellations and the stories that steer and inform us. Nighttime light pollution has a huge detrimental effect on migrating songbirds. Make sure your lights are aimed downward, which is a more effective lighting design and helps our winged relatives.

It is a beautiful reminder when you hear another person share their cultural history, oral traditions, and creation stories. It is a way of life, a deep understanding, the gift of existence in relationship with our home. I had not completely lost this link because as a child I was introduced to the Rooted Nations, my plant elders, who in unseen ways guided me toward this writing today.

One day while meditating in the forest, waiting to teach a class, this question arose: "What does it mean to be human?" How do we experience the richness, fullness of living, our full potential? How do we activate our own body's systems to flood ourselves with dopamine, serotonin, oxytocin, and all the other endocannabinoids that are part of this gift of the human experience? We are a living organism like all other organisms that response to Grandfather Sun and the water. Reclaiming our history helps us realign with our natural rhythms rather than the artificial environments we are existing in. Activating our own chemistry, our own pharmacology, being responsible for our own health and the health of our home, Mother Earth—that's reclamation.

PRINCIPLES OF KINSHIP

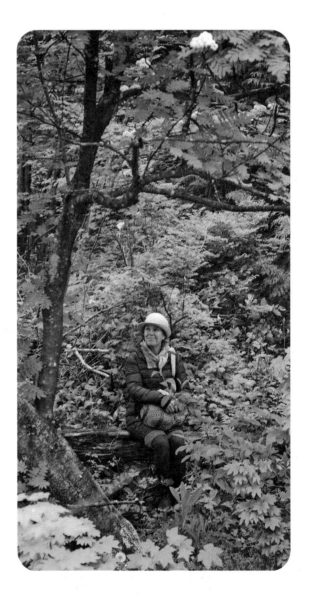

In a healing circle from many years ago, I learned how to speak of my relatives. The Rooted Nations, the Stone Nations, the Creepy Crawlers, the Ones-That-Fly, the Four-Leggeds, the Ones-That-Swim, and us, the Two-Leggeds, who come from the Star Nations. Ten years ago, I started teaching in our provincial school system about the Rooted Nations to help support and bring voice to Indigenous perspectives. The work of Kirkness and Barnhardt, 2001, in *Knowledge Across Cultures: A Contribution to Dialogue Among Civilizations*, wrote of responsibility, respect, relationship, reciprocity, and reverence. In First Peoples principles of learning and Indigenous ways of being, we observe a familiar interrelatedness of teachings that are not specific to any one Nation or Tribal society and that all follow a common thread. It is a road map, to be repeated over and over, as repetition anchors knowledge. A study of these five words in relation to the Rooted Nations follows.

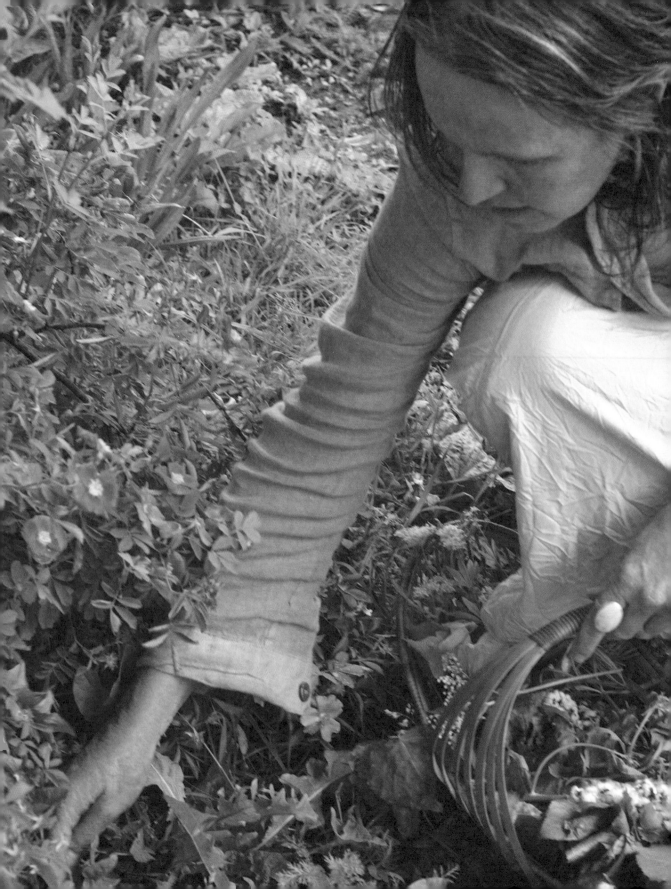

Responsibility
to Self and Others

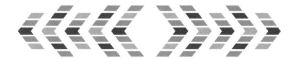

Re-spond-ability. Our ability to respond. Spoken in one of the four Métis language groups are the words of *pishkayimiwaan* (responsibility) and *nashkoomikoo* (to respond). In our Indigenous languages we are guided with the vibration of the words to walk in a good way with all of our relations, our relatives, and More-Than-Human-Kin. Indigenous language is the heart of culture, a way of being in a deep interconnectedness with the landscape and the gifts from Mother Earth.

Language arises from stillness and listening, expressing the aliveness that exists around us. Indigenous teachings are shared orally, with stories and metaphors, a collection of mostly verbs, "actions." English is predominately full of nouns, "things" that separate us from our responsibility and relationship with our kin. It is important to understand the essence of words for a greater understanding of cultures.

The etymology of *responsibility* defines the word as "answerable," "offered in return," from its Latin roots *respons*. Defining a quality or state of being, connected to morality, legal, or mental accountability, it is task-orientated. Responsibly is synonymous with "to care and protect."

This reminds me of the interconnectedness of Earth teachings—personal lived experiences, shared orally with stories and metaphors in an inclusive, wholistic approach. Within our ecosystems we discover that the living spirit resides in everything seen and unseen. There are no hierarchies; life is circular in an ever-flowing spiral like our Milky Way.

Reset, regenerate, and realign with the Original teachings that connect us to our heart. I am told the longest journey is from the mind to the heart. We are part of this intricate web. In the oral traditions, the land and the More-Than-Human-Kin guide us to live within the laws of nature, the Original instructions, the sacred laws. Let us make our decisions collaboratively for the future seven generations. The whole world is our family.

MUSINGS

Eco is Latin for "home," "household." Who lives in our household? We have a responsibility to improve relations with our living world, our home that is surrounding and supporting us. To live a good life with respect, humility, good hearts, and kindness.

Respect
the Law of Nature

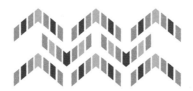

One cold day, I found a plump little caterpillar rolled up in a ball on my bedroom floor. I wonder why we naturally feel squeamish when touching insects? My first instinct was to use a tissue to pick her up, but I quickly opened myself up with courage to feel her on my skin. In my open hand, she unfurled and stretched her body. I found myself relating to her rolled-up posture, as we too roll up into a little ball when we need to feel safe. The moment she opened, I could feel her aliveness and I burst into tears. An overflowing, indescribable joy reverberated through my body, abounding with such reverence for her life. She started to crawl and explore. Then panic swept over me. What was I going to do with her? I thought about setting her in my garden of daffodils, hyacinth, and cyclamen, but realized she does not feed on introduced species. She needs the nourishment and shelter of native plants. Reluctantly, I placed her outside, knowing that there are no leaves on the ground in the manicured garden for her to burrow from the cold. I prayed that she would become food for the little chickadees, or that maybe someday she could become a butterfly; they are so scarce in this city, this place of sterility that we govern. In the landscape that surrounds me, I amplify my voice for all creatures to be heard: "Let us live so you can live."

Words hold power. The challenge with the diversity of languages is that it becomes more difficult to understand how others view and interact with the world. Speaking a language that is rooted in place speaks of the living world, reminding us that our kin are alive and we are all related.

The etymology of *respect*, a late middle English word, comes from the Latin *respectus*, from the verb *respicere: re*, meaning "back," and *specere*, meaning "look at." Look back at our ancient teachings. Let us consider, with reverence and admiration, how to honor and acknowledge the dignity of all life. It is not an intrinsic program to be respectful; it is a way of being that we must be taught. In relationship with others we build safety, trust, and mutual well-being. To be of service and model our love and care for others, we can start with active dialogue, collaboration, and listening.

In 2021, Suzanne Simard, PhD, launched her book, *Finding the Mother Tree.* In the beginning of her career she worked as a forester and was tasked with the challenge of understanding why the young plantings of new trees were not growing in our clear-cut logged forests. What Simard brought to the world's attention was the knowledge of the vast channels of communication and nutrient exchange that exist between the roots of the Mother Trees, the my-

MUSINGS

For so many reasons, we want to find evidence of munching insects in our gardens.

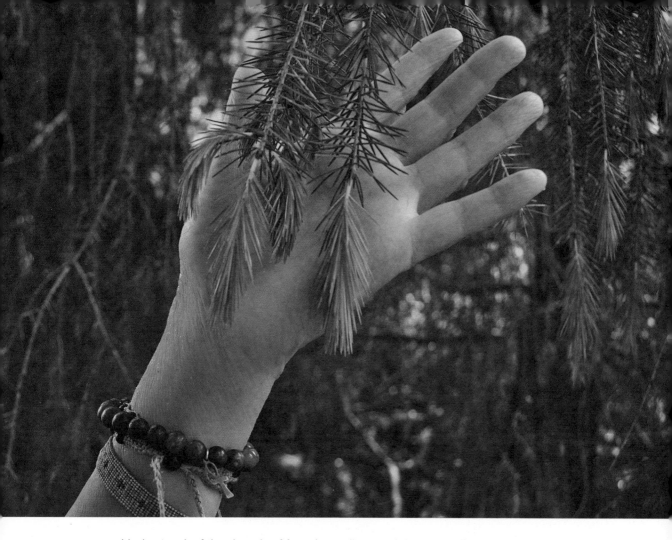

corrhizal network of tiny threads of fungal mycelium, and the tree's offspring. The mycorrhizal network transports water, nitrogen, carbon, and minerals to our More-Than-Human-Kin in an interconnected symbiotic relationship that includes a diversity of species living in the forest, both below and above ground. To be strong, healthy, and live long, the forest needs to be collaborative, to be altruistic, and to be generous. Here, too, are our instructions: Let us come together in a circle to dream, imagine, and reset our role together as the Two-Leggeds and consider what is possible for future generations.

When we pause and look back to our own history, we remember our relationship with Mother Earth and Father Sky. Let's reconcile with the lands and waters and replant what has been lost to support the wild that has a right to exist. Let us speak the language of the ancestors of the land we call our home and repair the relationship with our diverse human family.

In the physical act of generosity, we internally release dopamine, a neurotransmitter that makes us feel good.

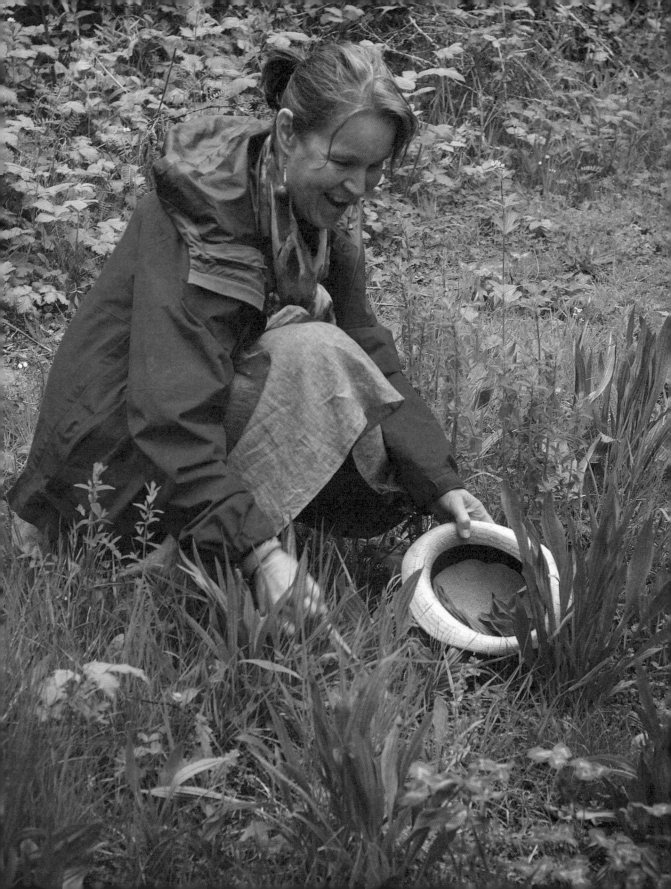

Relationship
to All That Exists

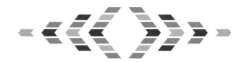

There was something magical about the year 2013. Robin Wall Kimmerer's book, *Braiding Sweetgrass*, was released, I started teaching children, and my dear friend, Lori Weidenhammer, received approval from the Vancouver Parks Board to plant a native Indigenous Medicine Wheel garden at one of our local parks. Most recreation spaces and public parks are curated with introduced species planted in isolation from each other. These beautiful but nonnative plants have not co-evolved with our Creepy Crawlers as our native Rooted Nations have. This was a groundbreaking act to reconcile with these lands.

A few years later I was asked to be the guardian of this little oasis called the Medicine Wheel Garden. It never ceases to amaze me how deeply this tiny parcel of a wild forest we created with the Rooted Nations supports life. It's a little ecosystem that supports a resident hummingbird, a multitude of other bird species, native bees, dragonflies, butterflies, beetles, worms, and so much more. The relationship building is slow, but we are grateful for the support of those who see a better future in our urban landscape. It's a participatory kinship, a relationship that is based in action.

Chief Charles Labrador of Acadia First Nations and Elder Albert Marshall, embraced a way of teaching that would become known by the Mi'kmaw word *etuaptmumk*—two-eyed seeing. It is a way to recognize there are many points of view and to learn how we can find the relational bridge that connects us regardless of our programs. Open one eye and see the world through the lens of Indigenous ways of knowing and then open the other eye to Western science. These are two views of inquiry and solutions, guiding values for intercultural collaboration, the gifts of a multitude of perspectives, shared principles, and remembering that there is only one planet. Don't we all want a future for our children? Let's see beyond.

To speak the truth and to reconcile, we have to concile first. We need open space to listen and reach across to make new friends and reclaim the relationship. The history of Indigenous medicine from this part of the world was shared with the settlers who arrived over five hundred years ago. We were responsible to share knowledge, help each other, and take care of our human family. There is an invisible thread that connects all of life that is relational. Be the model; lead for the unborn generations. If we don't teach right relations, who will?

Mino-bimaadiziwin, when activated, contains the present, the past, and the future. A good path, good life, good mind, good way, a worthwhile life, a long fulfilling life, our walk in life. It is a philosophical concept, rooted in Anishinaabe worldview as cited by artist Brent Debassige from the M'Chigeeng First Nations of Manitoulin Island, Ontario, Canada (2010) in the *Canadian Journal of Native Education*.

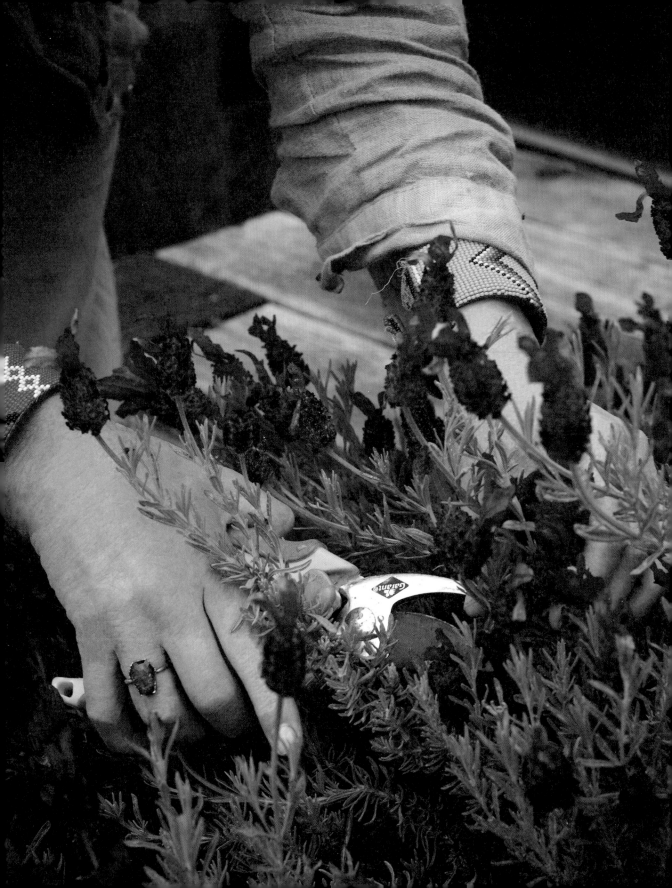

Reciprocity
and the Intersections of Giving

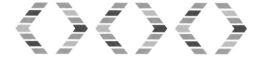

The sound of buzzing is an opportunity to slow down and witness the dancing and humming of bees, crawling and circling their little bodies around the inside of the pure beauty of a blooming flower. Intertwined in the dance is the joy of being present to the evolution in the interconnected-ness and the reciprocal exchange in process.

What is the practice? What are the instructions and how do we integrate the teaching of reciprocity? What rises up in our being when we experience the intersection of gift giving? How might we describe the deep gratitude, appreciation, and joy that unfold when this intersection occurs?

Our commitment, our assignment, our ONUS, is to plant the seeds from the gifts we receive and regenerate, to make space for all our relatives, and give thanks. Let us experience reciprocity as a physical act, not an intellectual concept. We are in an intricate dance in the web of life, and we have a relational obligation, task, and responsibility to foster life. A radical exchange of give and take, back and forth. The etymology of *re*, is "back," and *pro* is "forth." It is a participatory relationship with all that exists.

In our local schools, the children learn to say thank you in the Hunquminum language, spoken by the Musqueam People. It's a downriver dialect of the Halkomelem language. *Hy-chka* is "thank you," spoken to an individual. *Hy-sep-ka* is "thank you all." It's an invitation to speak to the Earth, the Mother, who will hear what was given to be spoken. To hear the language, the frequency, the melody, is a beautiful practice of back-and-forth reciprocity. It shows a deep appreciation for the Original inhabitants of place. I encourage you to reach out to the neighbors who hold the teachings and jump into the arena of relationship through reciprocity.

Reverence
for the Sacred Gift of Life

Bearing witness, devotion, humility, our reasons for waking in the morning—this is reverence. What is sacred in whose experience or through whose perception? Oral traditions are based on human experience and our relationship to Creation and living a peaceful coexistence with all things. The brilliance is our ability to grasp it and move with it. Our assignment is to understand and to integrate the experience.

A humble veneration of Creator's gift is alchemized through medicines and foods and so much more. It is Spirit who loves us and gives of their lives for us. Medicine is found where we live; our health is related to the Earth's health. Reverence is something greater than ourselves.

Our Turtle relatives have the ability to slow their heart rate down or even stop their heart rate for periods of time. Reptiles hibernate, known as brumation, for months without breathing in the mud. Turtles live slowly, breathe slowly, their hearts beat slowly, and they recover slowly and heal remarkably well when given time. When time is given with patience, Mother Earth heals. Our kin heal. We heal. Our devotion and commitment to repairing our ecosystems needs our attention.

In the living oral traditions of storytelling, there are various renditions of the creation story of Turtle Island, also known as North and Central America. Stories are transmissions, representing accumulated knowledge passed on through generations, filled with cultural values and the vision of the people who share the story. It is prayerful in nature, compelling us to walk in a good way. Through the repetition of listening, we are reminded again and again how to conduct ourselves. The stories from all over Turtle Island reach further back in time than the five hundred years of colonial history. These stories govern us, and, like everything that is alive, they are fluid. They assist us to transform our human condition, evolving life with the story.

Only recently have Creation stories been written to illuminate the supernatural into the wider world. The story of Sky Woman, who fell through a hole from Sky World, emphasizes the relationship to all the creatures of Creation who aid the new immigrant to this world. The community offers their many and various gifts to be of service for the pregnant Sky Woman, with her hands full of plants and medicines. A council is gathered to discuss and find ways to help the newcomer, and turtle

Storytelling shapes how we see and experience our world. It guides us so we won't forget how to participate in this ever-unfolding evolution of Mother Earth. Remember to remember cultural stories. Your family stories and the stories of the land you live upon.

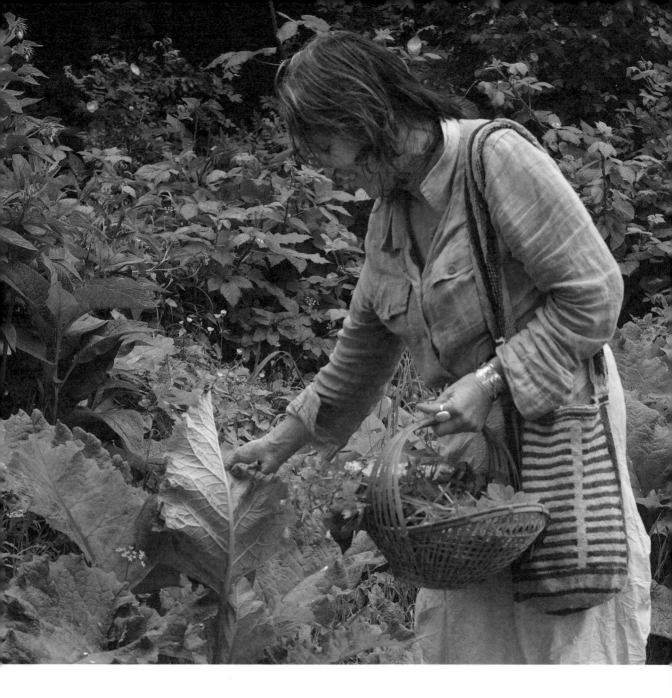

offers their back to co-create the foundation, the landscape to foster life. Many want to help. Each creature takes a turn to dive deep into the water to bring the mud (and its microorganisms) from the Ocean's floor, with no success. The smallest is little muskrat, who, with their will, commitment, and determination, surfaces with the mud as they succumb to their own life in reverence for the life of another and the life of the unborn. Sky Woman dances and sings her giving thanks songs, acknowledging the cycles of birth, life, death, and rebirth. As a good guest, she spreads the seeds and the wild plants take hold on the back of Turtle Island. The alchemy of everyone's contribution creates a diversity of life, celebrated and revered.

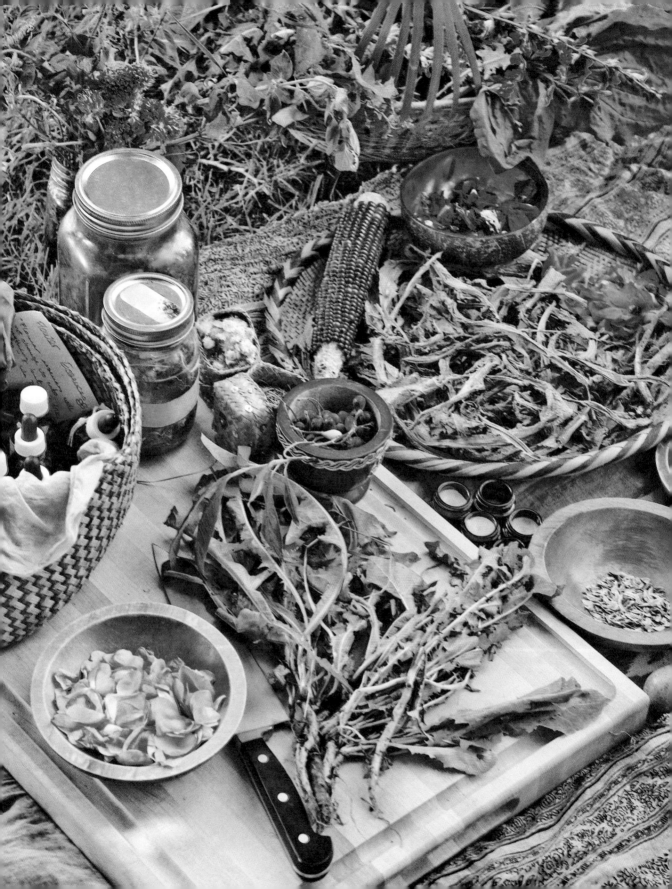

Honorable Harvest

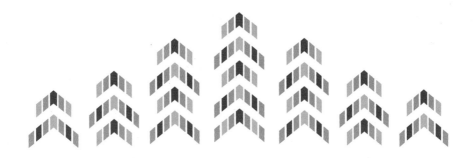

I learned about the honorable harvest from my teacher, Don Ollsin from Grassroots Herbalism. Pray and ask our Rooted Nations to reveal who holds the best medicine for those who are ill. Only take what you need. Ask for permission to the Rooted Nations and to the Original Guardians of the lands and waters. We don't want to break protocols or collect from sacred sites or break protocols that the Nations or Tribes have a deep relationship with. Sometimes you receive a "no;" trust that and walk away. But if you are given clearance, leave a sacred offering of other sacred medicines in exchange. I leave a strand of my hair, a prayer, a song sung out loud, or words spoken in the language of the land where I collect her gifts. I leave behind a physical offering so I remember how it feels for our relatives when we cut and uproot them.

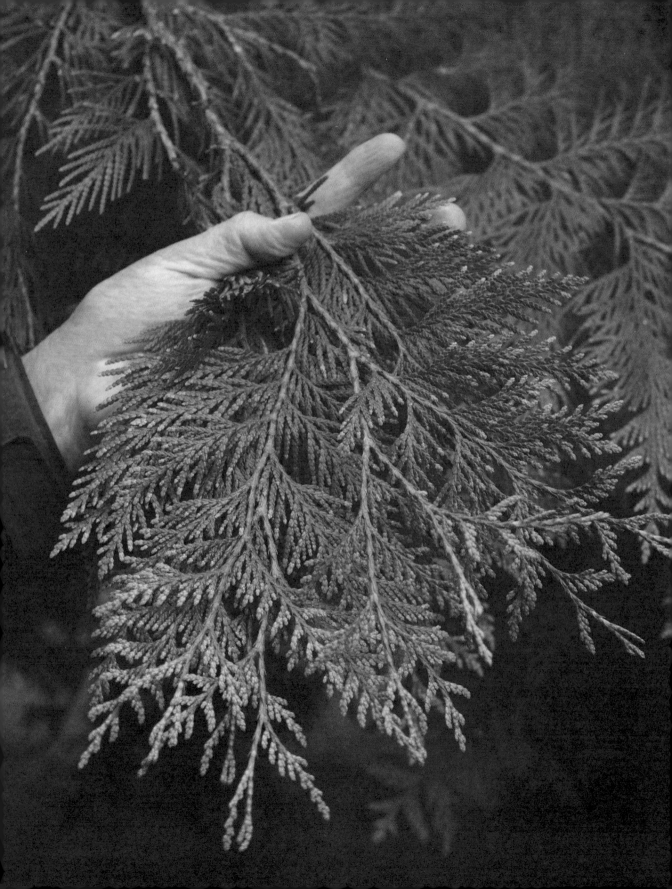

PART II

The Four Sacred Medicines

Indigenous traditions have a relationship with the plant's "vital spirit," who bestows their healing abilities when asked. Sacred is the celebration of life that gives up its life for our life. Sacred medicines are highly respected, linking us back in time to our ancestors and the original instructions. In "direct interrelationship between plants and people," it is not of the past, it is also the present. As we relearn about reciprocal exchange, we can ask how to navigate this deep link, to be still and listen. Our relationship with our More-Than-Human-Kin is not to treat them as commodities. It is a stewardship of agency. It is our obligation to reweave ourselves and walk in a good way and reenter the relationship. All cultures walked this way, while passing knowledge to our children.

Giving gifts, an exchange without expectations, is a sacred responsibility. The Rooted Nations offer their gifts in midwifery, in internal and external medicine, through steaming and sweat lodges, and to detoxify our bodies, minds, emotions, and malevolent spirits. The sacred medicines are honored during rituals and ceremonies, carrying prayers to Creator for protection. Physical health fails without the spiritual protocols of smudging, purging, prayers, dancing, and chanting.

It was uncommon for Indigenous People to experience cancer, tuberculosis, diabetes, or heart disease. It is different now, twenty-eight generations—five hundred years—later, compared to the twenty-five or thirty thousand years prior in which the Two-Leggeds cherished and respected the relationship with all of their relations. Our sovereignty was destroyed as we became dependent on the "new ways." Chief Seattle spoke of how, when his people had sugar, "the fight went out of them." I would say the same of all of us.

For centuries, every culture worldwide burnt herbs, roots, resins, and barks for cleansing, from frankincense and myrrh to rosemary to disinfect. Aromatic plants released a diverse repertoire of volatile oils to cleanse our body, mind, and spirit. Through the act of burning the physical matter, the rising smoke carries our prayers and intentions to the Spirit world for transformation.

MUSINGS

Like the Medicine Wheel teaching of the four directions, we are physical, mental, emotional, and spiritual. How do we balance these four directions daily?

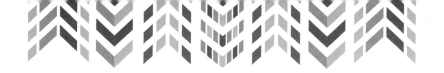

SAGE

Salvia apiana
Artemisia ludoviciana

Common names can vary from region to region, which is especially true for sage. Using botanical Latin binomial names allow us to differentiate between the true sages, those in the *Salvia* genus, and those in the *Artemisia* genus, which both refer to "sage" in the act of smudging. *Salvia* means to "save," "heal," or "redeem." It grows in poor soil conditions, often in deserts or high mountains, where it must adapt to thrive. The gift of pungent essential oil gives her protection from Grandfather Sun and is food for many animals. In the landscape, she offers wind cover for other relatives while her long taproot brings water to the surface for grasses and other herbs.

Sage's bitter flavor kick-starts the digestion, boosts the immune system, and calms the nerves. Her chemical constituents contain lactone glycosides of santonin and artemisinin, which are anthelmintic, powerful vermifuges to expel worms and intestinal parasites.

Salvia apiana

White sage was first threatened to extinction with the arrival of cattle back in the 1700s, but she is known to thrive in adverse conditions, including extreme heat and drought, even tolerating wildfires. She is a species that regenerates after fires, known as facultative seeders, which is important for pollinators. *Apiana*, meaning "belonging to the bees," has co-evolved with the bee genera of *Xylocopa* and *Bombus*, assisting in her gene production and diversity. She is under great threat from overharvesting, poaching, human activity, habitat encroachment, invasive species, and repeated wildfires and she needs us as guardians to protect her.

Artemisia

Of the four hundred species of *Artemisia*, these are the ones used medicinally: *Artemisia ludoviciana, A. nova, A. dracunculus, A. frigida, A. vulgaris, A. douglasiana*, and *A. tridentata*. Pinch and crush a small piece of the leaf to identify her resinous scent.

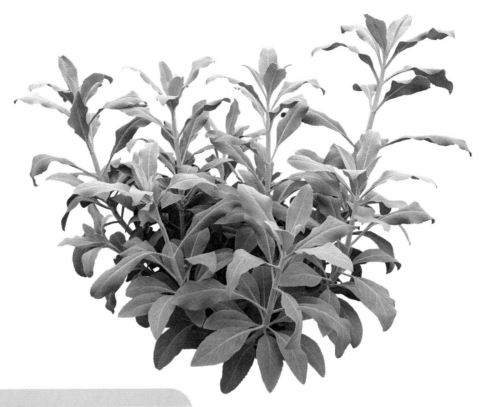

Make

Brew a strong tea, pour it into a spray bottle, and use as an insect repellent.

Cleansing

Burning leaves of white sage is a cultural sacred ceremony known as smudging. Recognized as an Indigenous purification ritual, offering up prayers, asking for guidance, connecting with Spirit, and releasing what no longer serves. Cleansing is practiced to gain the benefits of neutralizing airborne bacteria through the burning of sage varieties within the *Salvia* genus: *Salvia mellifera*, *Salvia officinalis*, *Salvia leucophylla*, and *Salvia clevelandii*.

Note

Sage contains thujone, a neurotoxin in large dosages.

White sage is deeply rooted in the traditions and spiritual practices of the Southern California Tribes of the Cahuilla, Chumash, Kumeyaay, Luiseno, and Tongva Peoples. As such, Indigenous gather white sage by leaving the roots and offering prayers of gratitude. When purchasing sage, consider whether the seller is in alignment with good ethical practices. You only need to burn a small leaf to receive the blessings.

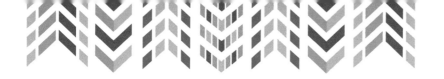

TOBACCO

Nicotiana rustica
Nicotiana glauca
Nicotiana clevelandii
Nicotiana longiflora
Nicotiana quadrivalvis
Nicotiana tobacum

Grandfather Tobacco is a potent herb, misunderstood and mistreated. Since time immemorial, she has been a sacred medicine. The ritual of breathing in and holding the smoke allows her to permeate and connect with all of life, and then we release her outward to the cosmos.

Professor Anne Charlton, in the article "Medicinal Use of Tobacco in History," published in the *Journal of the Royal Society of Medicine*, notes that the word *tobaco* or *tavaco* was used in reference to the vessel, a cane pipe, possibly made from elderberry stems, used by "Native Americans" for sniffing the tobacco smoke. The Kichaw and Shuar People of the South in Ecuador receive "tobacco wine" through the sinuses as the morning daylight breaks to acknowledge ancestors, praise the Creator's beauty, drink in the sunlight, and send prayers of healing with the sunbeams of Grandfather Sun. And to do the same again, when Grandfather Sun is in the west, setting.

Her other names include *petum, betum, cogioba, cohobba, quauhyetl, picietl* and *yietl*. The plant now classified in the *Nicotiana* genus has a variety of species and names recorded in older pharmacopoeias. The Anishinaabe People refer to her as *asemaa*.

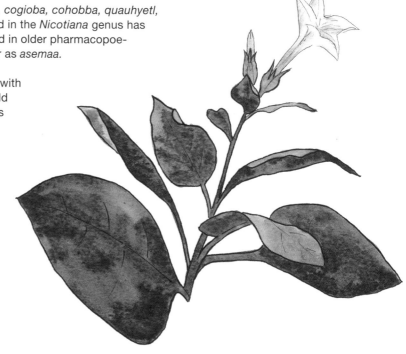

Columbus brought home this new herb with high hopes in Europe that tobacco would be the panacea to many ailments. It was referred to as the "holy herb" or "God's remedy." Around the 1500s, it was observed by explorers that tobacco was mixed with lime or chalk to whiten the teeth, a practice that still exists in India, where commercial toothpaste contains powdered tobacco known as *masheri*.

Tobacco leaves contain alkaloids of harmala and nicotine, as well as anatabine and anabasine, which in low dosages is a stimulant, in high dosages a depressant. The roots produce pyridine and pyrrolidine, and together produce nicotine, which is addictive. How nicotine enters the body (through the lungs, mouth, or skin) impacts the speed and intensity of nicotine entering the blood. Smoking it takes about ten seconds to reach the brain versus an hour with a nicotine patch.

Inside the brain, nicotine binds to nicotinic acetylcholine receptors located on nerve cells, causing the release of dopamine, GABA, glutamate, acetylcholine, and nor-adrenaline, which affect brain function and physiological systems throughout the body. Here on Turtle Island, the people have been growing and using tobacco long before the Europeans arrived, experiencing her pleasurable effects and treatment of illnesses.

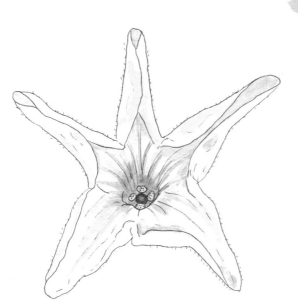

Note

It is poisonous to eat the leaves.

Make

Breathe in the fresh leaves to expel persistent headaches, relieve cold symptoms, and ease pain. Make a juice to treat ulcerated abscesses, sores, and diarrhea; it is also a narcotic. Apply powdered tobacco to heal wounds and burns.

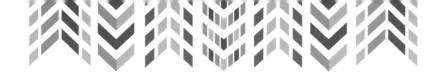

SWEETGRASS

Hierochloe alpina
Hierochloe occidentalis
Hierochloe odorata

Lyinikaysowin is a Cree teaching that reminds us "you know how to make yourself strong." Within the whole community of species who all live together in a balanced reciprocal relationship, protocols exist to keep the balance intact for self-sustenance. This teaching is integral to contributing, participating, and knowing our role in that balance.

Indigenous knowledge and traditions are tied directly to the landscape. Before the settlers arrived, more than five hundred languages were spoken, representing distinct cultures. For thousands of years this "lifestyle and library," as stated in Enrique Salmon's book *Iwigara: The Kinship of Plants and People*, ecological knowledge overlaid within the ecosystem and landscapes, were sustainable and well managed, and still are when given the space with applied local teachings.

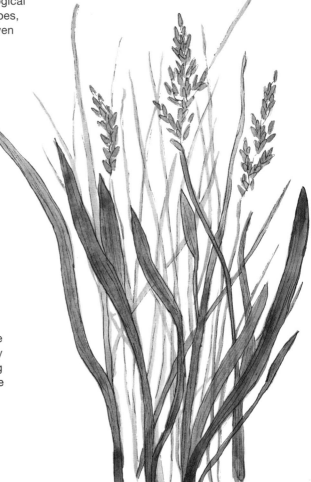

As a hardy circumpolar species with a rhizomatous root system, sweetgrass, a perennial, is known as holy grass in Europe. The Greek *hierochloe* means "holy grass," and *odorata* means "fragrant." This fragrant holy grass was laid in front of church doorways, for sweetgrass's aroma to be trodden upon. In France, she was made into candy, used to flavor tobacco and soft drinks, and added to perfumes. In Russian, the plant added flavor to teas. The Sami People of the Scandinavian regions braided and dried it for perfume and stored it in clothing. Here on Turtle Island she is a ceremonial holy purifier, incense, medicine, and perfume and is woven into baskets.

Sweetgrass grows a culm up to 3 feet (91 cm) tall that is often reddish-purple at the base. She prefers prairie grasslands, subalpine meadows, wetlands, sloughs, and stream banks. To tend sweetgrass, we need to balance overharvesting and underharvesting. With grasses, they adjust to disturbances. How do we adjust to the changing times? By understanding and following how to be in the symbiotic dance with Creation, with medicine, with life.

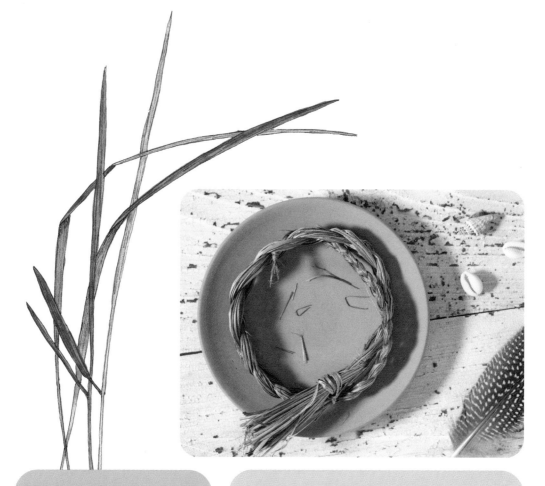

Note

Sweetgrass contains phytol, which repels mosquitoes, and the sweet vanilla aroma of coumarin, which is known to thin our blood when consumed.

Harvest

Leave a gift of gratitude to our relatives, ask permission, never take some from the first patch found and take only what you need. When we respect our More-Than-Human-Kin, they flourish. And let others know you have been in the patch by tying a little ribbon in the area so they won't come in and collect more.

To braid sweetgrass, first offer your gratitude and set intentions. Gather seven strands for each bundle. The first bundle of seven strands reminds us of the seven generations who came before us; the second bundle represents the seven sacred teachings of love, wisdom, respect, honesty, courage, truth, and humility; and the last bundle stands for the seven generations to come after you. Finally, braid the three bundles together with good words and let dry before burning to send up your prayers to Creator.

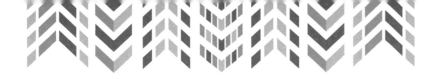

CEDAR

Thuja plicata
Thuja occidentalis

I grew up with western red cedar and I have been blessed to sit with her, a Grandmother over 1,200 years old, 200 feet (61 m) high. She can photosynthesize in poor sunlight and has a wide, shallow root system. When these trees are growing here in the city, the grass growing under her skirt is competing with the dwindling yearly rainfall and many Grandmothers are dying.

The word *cedar* describes "wood" from a number of conifers that yield fragrant, durable timber. True cedars, native to the Mediterranean and the Himalayans, are classified in the Pinaceae family, genus *Cedrus*. Their evergreen needles grow in clusters, and the fat female cones grow upright. False cedars reside in the Cupressaceae family, with the genera of *Calocedrus, Chamaecyparis, Juniperus*, and *Thuja*. Leaves are scaly and fanlike, and the female cones are very small. The bark is often reddish and stringy; it peels off relatively easy. Distinct differences allows us to tell true cedar from false cedar, which are native to East Asia and Turtle Island.

Thuja occidentalis, also known as eastern arborvitae and *Thuja plicata*, western red cedar, are both considered the Tree of Life. Both are highly revered, an important relationship that offers many gifts for the First Peoples to survive and thrive. In the east, she symbolizes the balance between the Two-Leggeds and the rest of Creation, and sending prayers to Grandmother Cedar will open up communication with the unseen.

Joseph Pitawanakwat, an Anishinaabe plant medicine educator, speaks of *Thuja occidentalis*'s ability to collect garbage; it opens the sweat glands to expel the toxins out through the skin, to avoid taxing the kidneys and liver. It supports the immune system, utilizes energy, and helps slow the aging process.

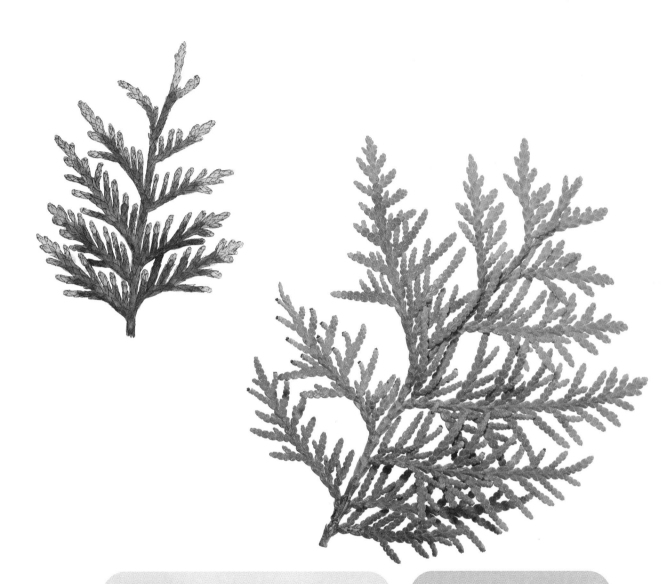

Make

Grandmother Cedar is a stimulant and emollient for the skin. Add one part chopped herb to two parts oil, infuse for 4 weeks, strain, and apply it topically as an antibacterial and antifungal. Our sacred cedar can also be served as a tea when gathering. Infuse cedar in apple cider vinegar as a wart medicine. A cedar steam with her boughs will help with colds, coughs, and stuffy noses.

Note

Cedar contains a terpene, thujone, which interacts with fat and is not water-soluble. It is reported that you can drink it daily in moderate amounts. Do not use when pregnant or with kidney challenges. Sacred medicines are potent and should be used under the guidance of an Elder.

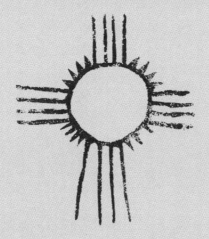

The Four Seasons of Wild, Native, and Medicinal Plants

Nature's pattern is the rhythmic shifting yet continuous cycles of seasons, of birth, life, death, and rebirth. Nature is chaotic and then order is restored. Reflected in this natural pattern is us, as we are nature. The perpetual gifts of nature's patterns influence our internal clock, which is activated through sunlight. Grandfather Sun's rays stimulate the production of serotonin, a chemical messenger that is transmitting and communicating information throughout our bodies. The early morning blue spectrum of sunlight hits our eyes, activating serotonin, which helps wake us up. This process in our brain releases a cascade of hormones, turning on our internal systems and moving our brain waves from the delta (the dreaming state) to the theta, alpha, and then beta phases (our waking state). In the evening, the process reverses when the red spectrum light hits our eyes, as Grandfather Sun sets in the west. The pineal gland transmutes serotonin into melatonin, slowing down our brain waves. We start an inward journey to rest, relax, and let go of the day, slipping into the quiet and stillness where we can now fall asleep. Known as the circadian rhythm, this cycle is similar to the changing seasons throughout the year. When we move out of this natural cycle we become out of balance.

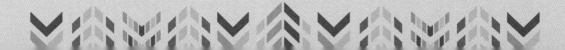

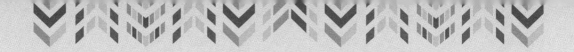

For the Rooted Nations, Grandfather's rays activate plant hormones like auxin, which helps our More-Than-Human-Kin grow toward the sunlight. Plants give their gifts of nourishment, a diversity of flavors and textures, medicines that range from gentle to deadly, natural dyes, materials to weave and make textiles. Pollen, along with nectar, nourish other living creatures through the variety of vitamins and minerals found within the Rooted Nations. Like all life, plants die and then eventually decompose to regenerate the cycle again and again. Through my own experience walking the land, asking questions, and seeking guidance to have a better understanding and deeper relationships, the Rooted Nations have led me to a greater awareness and appreciation of my own body's wisdom.

With the tilting of Mother Earth and the rising of Grandfather Sun, we witness the activation of so many creatures in this cycle of life. In ancient cultures worldwide, humans created physical markers to acknowledge the movement of Grandfather Sun, like the famous Stonehenge, Newgrange, Chichén Itzá, Machu Picchu, and here on Turtle Island, Chaco Canyon, to name a few. Today as I write, we have just passed the midway point between the winter solstice and the spring equinox, a time when many cultures still honor traditions, including the Celtic Imbolc and Candlemas, a Christian celebration. At this time, our ancestors would gather in community and call in the guidance and intelligence of the community for the forthcoming season. We would celebrate with prayers and rituals, feasting on last winter's harvest, dancing and singing into the night around bonfires. We would ask the ones who came before us how to carefully prepare the land. We would sing to the sleeping seeds to awaken, to bring us life as Mother Earth warms her womb to receive the seeds and continue the cycle for the next generations.

As people, we have always recycled our waste back into the system to feed the microorganisms that live in the soil. Amoebas, protozoa, fungi, nematodes, and bacteria live there, along with so much more. These microscopic organisms are integral to good soil health and assist in growing strong, healthy Rooted Nations that feed and nourish us. There is so much to explore in learning about soil health and many ways to support it, in addition to reintroducing ourselves back into its service and contributing once again to our role in assisting the cycles. Compost your kitchen scraps, feed the soil aged manure, leave the leaves on Mother Earth, collect the water. Acknowledge your good contribution. Go outside, sit, enjoy, and witness the abundance of life.

We recently had a cold spell, and our once yearly snowfall impacted many of our introduced ornamental plants as they either dropped their leaves or died. As I was out wandering and witnessing, I wondered what might the Rooted Nations be communicating? Could they be asking us to understand the teaching, and what might we be doing (or not doing) to help the Rooted Nations? Could we consider leaving the leaves on the ground, to blanket Mother Earth, to keep the roots warm, to create homes for a diversity of insects, to hold the water moisture? And the little caterpillar I found, she will now be able to burrow under the piles of leaves where our native birds find food to feed their baby chicks in the spring.

Nature is always speaking to us in this ancient communication. Our Indigenous brothers and sisters have been listening for time immemorial. Be like the forest and leave the leaves, rake them into your garden beds, and while you move your body, you will have an opportunity to listen. What do you hear and what do you not hear? Touch base with yourself, as nature heals.

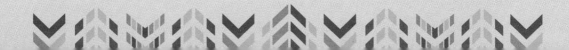

DANDELION

Taraxacum officinale

A cultural food, dandelion is known as a pioneer plant, and her seeds travel up to 5 miles (8 km). She grows quickly in disturbed areas to cover and protect the soil while becoming home to countless insects. Dandelion teaches us how to be a good guest, as she makes space for diversity of life by offering food, medicine, dyes, shade, and craft supplies, all while remineralizing the soil and feeding microorganisms. One of the first to show up in the spring, her bright, yellow flowers, full of pollen and nectar, provide nourishment to insects and hummingbirds.

Another exceptional attribute is that the whole plant is a complete protein. Her blossoms, leaves, stems, and roots are all edible and medicinal.

NOTE

Avoid if you have bleeding disorders or allergies to ragweed or latex. Do not use over a long period of time. Dandelion is a diuretic, so we do not want to flush the kidneys for too long. Instead, dose one week on, one week off.

Dandelion is a great teacher for our children to witness the unfolding of three celestial bodies during different phases of the dandelion's life cycle. The bright yellow flower reflects our Grandfather Sun. The puffball sphere full of seeds reminds us of Grandmother Moon, and when we blow the seeds, they become stars, dispersing for more relatives to grow. We, too, migrate like the seeds.

Flowers

The spring flowers release a subtly sweet, bitter-tasting flavor and the leaves, stems, and roots are bitter. Bitters are one of the energetics of plants that activates bile production, which helps in the breakdown of fats and improves digestion. It also creates healthy muscles, tones the internal organs, and assists with greater strength and stamina. Dandelion oxygenates and purifies the blood through alkalizing the body and regenerating cellular integrity.

Lecithin is a chemical compound belonging to a group of phospholipids. These lipids are important for the brain, blood, nerves, and other tissues. Dandelion pollen contains B vitamins, protein, amino acids, and trace minerals. Coumestrol is a plant estrogen found in her flowers and stems. It can help balance our hormones and activate breast milk production.

MAKE: Stir-fry the stems with butter and garlic, and scramble your eggs into the mixture. You can also use the flowers in jellies, pancakes, or cookies, or scatter the petals on cupcakes. Ferment dandelion flowers to brew wine. For topical application, infuse dandelion roots and flowers in oil. Use for massaging sore muscles or massage into breasts to move toxins and assist in dissolving cysts.

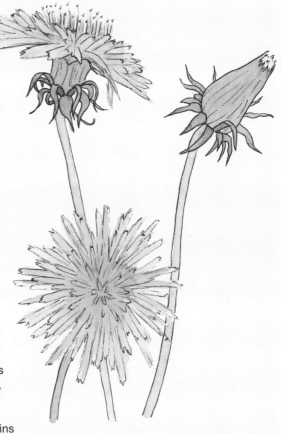

continued on next page

Root

Dandelion root is a nutritive that helps replenish the blood. It is rich in iron, calcium, beta-carotene, pectin, and inulin. Iron attaches to oxygen, supporting anemia, and assists with the production of dopamine. Beta-carotene converts in the small intestine to vitamin A, an important vitamin to keep the eyes healthy and to build strong cell walls, so pathogens like bacteria and viruses are more challenged to enter the cell. Pectin helps prevent constipation and encourages beneficial flora to thrive in the colon, eliminating unfriendly bacteria and pulling toxins out.

Collect the root in early spring for higher glucose levels; harvest in the autumn for higher starches and inulin. These carbohydrates, the fructans and starches, help balance blood sugars. The inulin is a low-glycemic soluble fiber and not absorbed in the gastrointestinal tract. As dandelion root ferments in the large intestine, it feeds countless bacteria and other microorganisms, creating a healthy gut pH. Some of these bacteria are used by the liver for energy production. Flatulence, bloating, belching, cramping, and diarrhea are indicators of an unbalanced gut biome.

MAKE: Make an apple cider vinegar tincture with one part dried root into two parts apple cider vinegar. Let sit for 4 weeks, strain, and use for salad dressings, marinades, or drink 1 teaspoon in 1 cup (240 ml) of water 30 minutes before meals. Her root can be stored in the freezer or dried to rehydrate in soups.

Leaves

Collect her leaves in the early spring, before she flowers, as they are less bitter tasting and receive the earth's minerals. Potassium balances the cell's sodium levels, flushes the kidneys, and lowers stress that can be caused by low potassium levels. Magnesium helps rebuild the blood and alleviates bad breath. Other minerals give strength, increase bone density, and inhibit the buildup of plaque on our teeth. Vitamin C is known to support the immune system, offers energy, and is one of the building blocks to create connective tissues like collagen, supporting good heart health. Vitamin K helps eliminate the excessive buildup of acidic crystals that can contribute to gout. It also helps with postpartum bleeding and generally helps the blood clot.

MAKE: Make salads, stir-fries, smoothies, egg dishes, lasagna, and pesto with her young leaves. Use her in a juice fast for rheumatism or arthritis, twice daily. For a spring cleanse, eat dandelion greens with apples or lemons for 3 to 7 days. Add ginger if you need some heat.

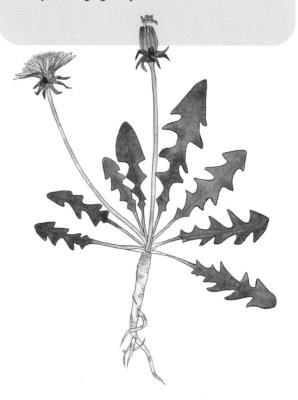

PLANTAIN

Plantago major
Plantago lanceolata

The leaf of *Plantago major*, known as frog's leaf here in the Pacific Northwest, has a similar shape to the green frog that was prevalent in our surrounding forest and marsh areas. As a child, I would find those little kin when I went out scouting for life. Frog's leaf is an annual visitor originally from Asia via the Mediterranean and North Africa. Referred to as "white man's footprint," she was carried by new immigrants to Turtle Island in the 1600s. Her abundant seeds would populate wherever newcomers walked, found commonly in schoolyards and on the edges of frequently walked paths. *Plantago lanceolata* is a long leaf plantain also known as ribwort.

Plantain is in the same family as *Plantago ovata*, which produces psyllium husks, helpful for digestion and moving the bowels. She contains vitamins A, C, and K, and potassium along with soluble and insoluble fiber for digestive health. She is highly absorbent of moisture, so consume lots of water to avoid digestive distress like gas, bloating, or constipation.

Make

Plantain is a fresh addition to salads and other green dishes. Easy to eat, it's delicious and green tasting. Add it to soups, green drinks, and pesto. Older plantain leaves are best cooked. The plant enzymes neutralize bee stings as well as mosquito and spider bites. Make a poultice by chewing rolled-up fresh leaves and applying it to an insect bite. Plantain is also antimicrobial. A tea, poured into a spray bottle and spritzed onto your tongue, can help with smoking cravings. Chew on the root for toothaches. An alcohol tincture with one part dried plant material to two parts alcohol is effective for bladder and urinary tract infections. Plantain is helpful as a bowel cleanser: soak the autumn seeds in clean water, drink fresh water first, and then drink the soaked seeds.

CHICKWEED

Stellaria media

Showing up early in the New Year or even the last calendar months, chickweed responds to Grandfather Sun. Ancient Romans called her the "elixir of life." With cool weather and the right conditions, little ecosystems are created around our landscape and give us flavorful food with more nutrition. She is a living mulch that protects the soil biome of nematodes, protozoas, bacteria, and fungi that are interacting with the plants to support the growth of our foods. She is cooling, demulcent, and expectorant; relieves coughs, and is an ally externally for skin disease and itching as she is anti-inflammatory. Chickweed is full of vitamins A, and C, iron, zinc, calcium, potassium, copper, magnesium, manganese, niacin, phosphorus. She is great for digestion as she contains saponins, which help regulate the gut flora, absorb toxins, and are eliminated through the bowels. She also helps dissolve fat cells and lowers cholesterol. The energetics of chickweed is cooling for the body. She is often recommended for bladder, kidney, and urinary tract infections. Chickweed infused in oil helps inflamed, itchy skin and can assist with acne and rosacea.

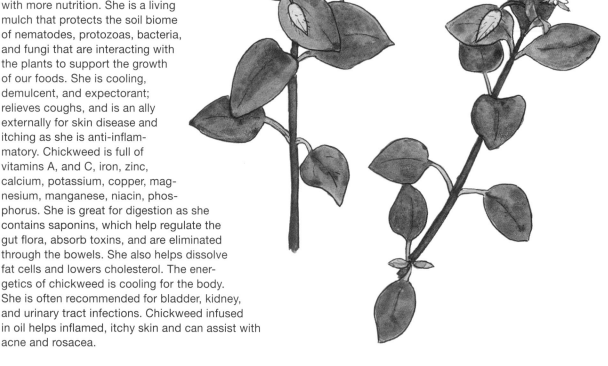

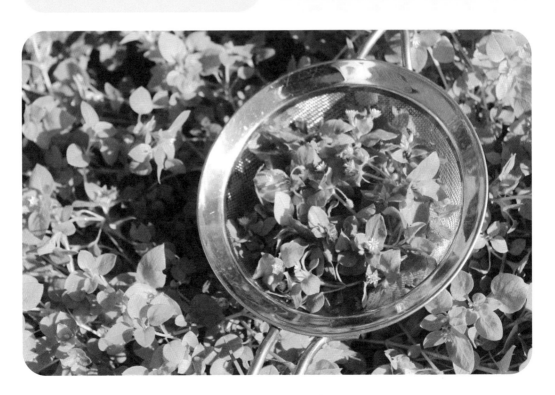

Make

Add chickweed fresh to salads, soups, omelets, quiches, and green drinks. Cook by boiling for 5 minutes and serving with butter. Add seeds to muffins or trail mix. In a blender, make a green dip with chickweed, garlic, olive oil, salt, and apple cider vinegar. As a tincture, use alcohol instead of vinegar for a longer shelf life. Juice the fresh plant and take 1 to 3 teaspoons three times daily.

Look-alikes

Scarlet pimpernel (*Anagallis arvensis*), sometimes called poison chickweed, is known to be toxic. Scarlet pimpernel is covered with hair all over the leaves and stems. Chickweed, however, has a little hair on only one side of her stem.

CURLY DOCK

Rumex crispus

Also known as yellow dock from the plant family of Polygonaceae, the buckwheat family, she is a native from Europe and western Asia. From our ancient traditions from Europe, spiritually yellow dock has been said to clear the blockages that prevent one from moving forward. Yellow dock helps release emotions and anxiety intertwined with the past, or old pain. She supports transitions in life as you transform into new phases.

Curly dock grows from 3 to 6 feet (1 to 1.8 m) in height, with narrow, slender, light green, curled-edge leaves. Broadleaf dock, *Rumex obtusifolius*, has a 4-inch (10 cm) wide basal, shield-shaped leaf at the bottom of the stalk, whereas the curly dock leaf is only 1 inch (2.5 cm) across and shaped like a sword. The young leaves in early spring, stalks, and seeds are all edible. She has a long flowering stage from June to September. To help stop the spread of seeds, harvest before she goes to seed or collect the seeds before the Ones-That-Fly do.

Due to the oxalate and tannin content, she should not be consumed by folks with endometriosis, hemorrhoids, any intestinal obstruction, unknown abdominal pain, or nephropathy. Consume with caution as she contains anthraquinones, aromatic organic compounds that have been used as laxatives and have antimicrobial, anti-inflammatory, and potent anticancer properties. We find these compounds in various plants like rhubarb, buckthorn, aloe vera, cascara, and senna leaf.

This medicine is helpful in small amounts as a laxative and used only for short periods of time. Slightly larger amounts can cause diarrhea as curly dock works to stimulate peristalsis, our intestinal mobility beginning in the pharynx, contracting and relaxing longitudinal and circular muscles. She moves food out through the bowels as she increases mucus production and the secretion of water in the colon. Curly dock can be helpful for unbalanced menstrual cycles. She is a diuretic, helping with water retention when the bladder is inflamed and when there are urinary stones. This is a natural cleanser for the liver, spleen, kidneys, and bladder.

Topically, the crushed leaf can neutralize the sting of stinging nettle. Harvest her spindled-shaped, deep yellow root and rhizome root in the early spring before she puts out leaves. The yellow root is high in iron and might be helpful instead of iron supplements, which can be constipating. Some reports mention that if she is overconsumed she may cause colon cancer. She is not advised for anyone with kidney or liver disorders, gout, or arthritis or is breastfeeding.

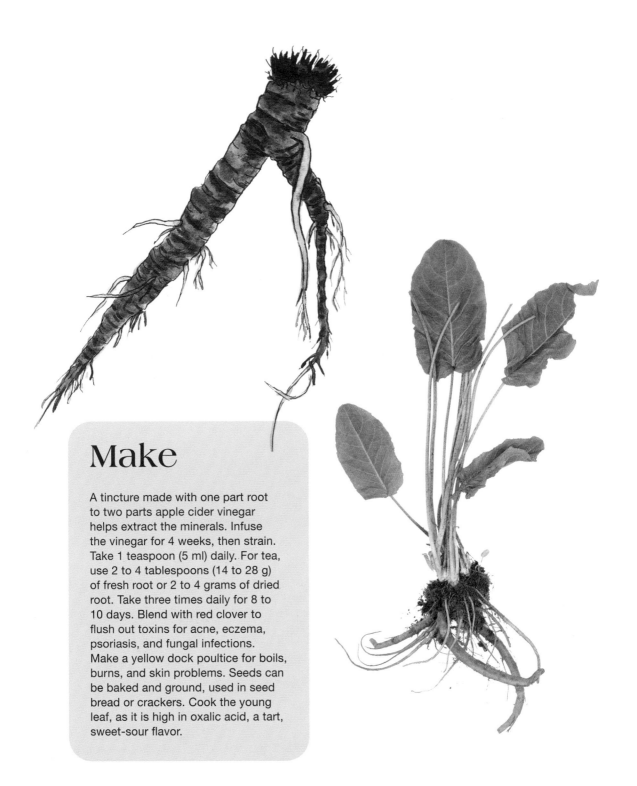

Make

A tincture made with one part root to two parts apple cider vinegar helps extract the minerals. Infuse the vinegar for 4 weeks, then strain. Take 1 teaspoon (5 ml) daily. For tea, use 2 to 4 tablespoons (14 to 28 g) of fresh root or 2 to 4 grams of dried root. Take three times daily for 8 to 10 days. Blend with red clover to flush out toxins for acne, eczema, psoriasis, and fungal infections. Make a yellow dock poultice for boils, burns, and skin problems. Seeds can be baked and ground, used in seed bread or crackers. Cook the young leaf, as it is high in oxalic acid, a tart, sweet-sour flavor.

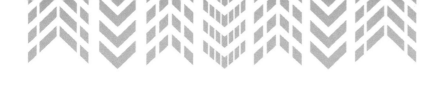

EVERGREEN TIPS

Hemlock: *Tsuga*
Fir: *Abies*
Spruce: *Picea*
Pine: *Pinus*
Douglas Fir: *Pseudotsuga*

When the colonists arrived to the east shores of Turtle Island they were served pine needle tea to treat scurvy, a disease caused by a lack of nutrition, specifically vitamin C. When you taste any of the needles from evergreens, you'll immediately recognize the zesty, citrus flavor that indicates they are full of vitamin C. Each species of evergreen has a slightly different flavor profile for sourness. Taste them all and see which tip resonates with you. Fresh spring tips taste the best.

In the late spring, look for evergreen trees for the new, bright-green needle growth. The tips can be eaten fresh, made into tea, or dried for a few days, then infused in honey or vodka. Take care not to harvest from the terminal bud, as that contributes to the elongation of the main branch. Consider collecting after windstorms have brought the branches to the forest floor to see what has been made available from our Rooted Nations. Plants are sentient like us and feel when we cut, clip, pull, and pinch off her growth. Be mindful to take only what you need.

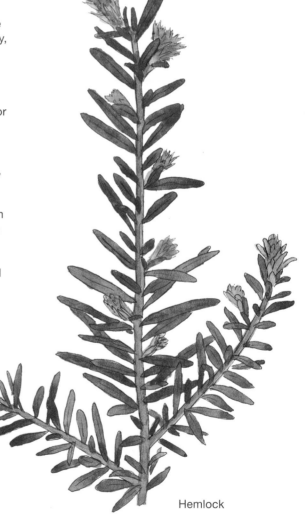

Hemlock

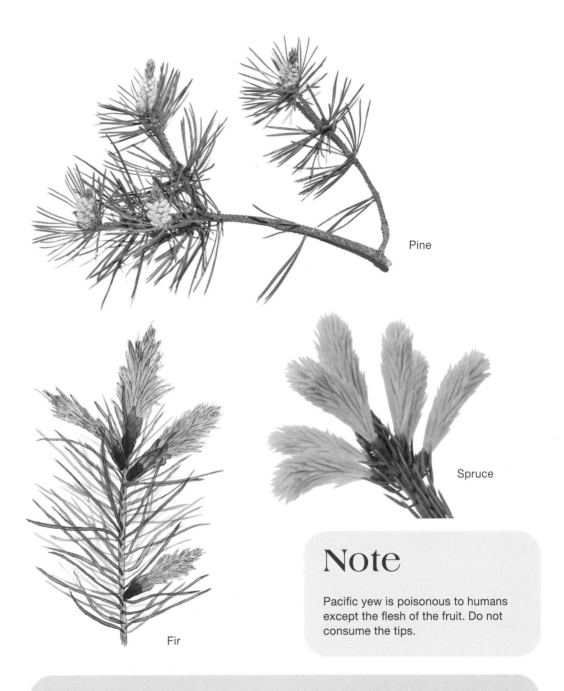

Pine

Spruce

Fir

Note

Pacific yew is poisonous to humans except the flesh of the fruit. Do not consume the tips.

Susun Weed, a folklore herbalist from the East Coast, has been teaching for over five decades. She shares a recipe for pine needles infused in apple cider vinegar. Use either white pine (*Pinus strobus*) or pinyon pine (*P. edulis*), as these white pines hold a more flavorful aroma, like balsamic vinegar. The hard pines like *P. radiata* and *P. ponderosa* have more pitch and taste like turpentine. Infuse for 4 to 6 weeks.

STINGING NETTLE

Urtica dioica

Stinging nettle is one of the most nutritive herbs on the planet. She has many gifts from the leaves, roots, and seeds. In late winter, after the midway point of Imbolc, a Celtic festival acknowledging the awakening of Mother Earth, we can witness her emerging tips poking through the leaf litter. Stinging nettle loves decaying leaves, moist soil, and cow pastures.

Nettle leaf is a safe cleansing herb and can be super helpful for chronic disorders that require long-term treatment. She is high in chlorophyll, histamine, iron, calcium, silica, zinc, carotenes, phytosterols, antioxidants, magnesium, potassium, boron, manganese, selenium, sulfur, and vitamins A, B, C, and K. Nettles gently stimulates the lymphatic system, helping remove waste from our body. She also stimulates breast milk production. Stinging nettle leaf, like dandelion leaf, promotes the elimination of uric acid from our joints, which irritates arthritis. She stops inflammation, excretes waste, and aids in bone remineralization. Nettles soothe gastrointestinal symptoms, hay fever, enlarged prostate, hemorrhoids, menstrual symptoms, and uterine fibroids. Gather the protein-rich seeds in late summer to add to breads. Harvest the roots, which are helpful for benign prostate hyperplasia, in the fall through to the spring.

Stinging nettle rebuilds the adrenal glands, supports the kidneys, is great for bone health, and reduces stress. She is a blood purifier, rejuvenates our energy, enhances the immune system, improves the thyroid, complements chemotherapy, and acts as a mild laxative and diuretic along with other amazing gifts. Traditionally, the antibacterial and mold-resistant stalks were harvested in late fall and made into fiber for fishing nets around the world.

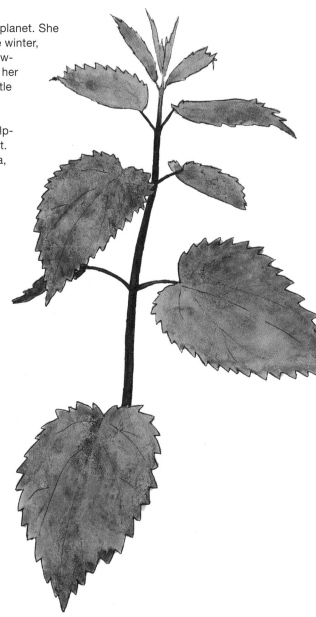

Collect the leaves in the early spring and don't fear the sting! The stinging barbs are full of formic acid, which is believed to help release serotonin. You can, however use plantain or dock to neutralize the sting. She loses her sting when she starts to wilt or after she has been blended or cooked. If you are histamine intolerant, you will not be able to use stinging nettle. Collect her regularly until she flowers, as the surface cells of her leaves produce cystolith crystals. The epidermal cell walls form deposits of calcium carbonate that are irritating to the kidneys. This evolution may have come about to stop our animal kin from eating her before she produces the seeds.

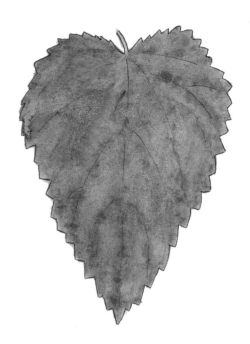

Make

Add nettles to any recipe that calls for greens such as spinach or kale. Add to soups, stews, lasagna, quiche, pesto, teas, and spanakopita. You can also substitute stinging nettles for any other wild greens in a recipe. When adding nettles to your soup, cook each day you warm up the leftovers to extract more minerals. An overnight decoction allows her medicine to release the kaleidoscope of minerals and vitamins. For allergies, make an alcohol tincture with one part leaf to two parts alcohol and steep for 30 days. Take 20 to 60 drops twice daily. An apple cider tincture can be used in salad dressings or marinades, or you can drink 1 teaspoon (5 ml) 30 minutes before meals to activate the digestive tract.

CLEAVERS

Galium aparine

Have you ever noticed when walking in a dense mass of vegetation that you get caught by a clinging stalk, with six to eight tiny hooked and prickled leaves whirling around on a long, slightly square stem? This is cleavers. She loves moist areas, often near bodies of water, and climbing over other plants. You can identify her by pinching off a stem and placing it on your body, as she will cling to your clothes.

Cleavers leaves, stems, and seeds are edible and collected in the early spring. With this wild spring food we notice more subtle, slightly fresh, green, sweet notes of cucumber, green pea, or even honeydew in her flavor. Cleavers contains coumarin, the glycoside asperuloside, and tannins. She is a soothing and relaxing diuretic, mild astringent, and mild diaphoretic, which helps you sweat to release fluids. She is known for her support of the lymphatic system. She breaks up congestion, especially in the pelvis, and is a demulcent for the urinary tract when you are experiencing cystitis, urethritis, prostatitis, or pyelonephritis. Cleavers are good for reducing edema caused by water retention of kidney origins. She is very helpful for dry skin like eczema and psoriasis. There are no known toxic effects on the central nervous system or gastrointestinal tract with cleavers.

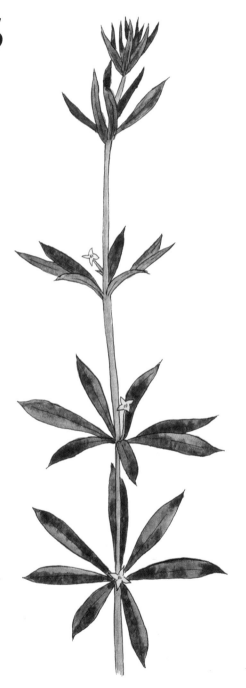

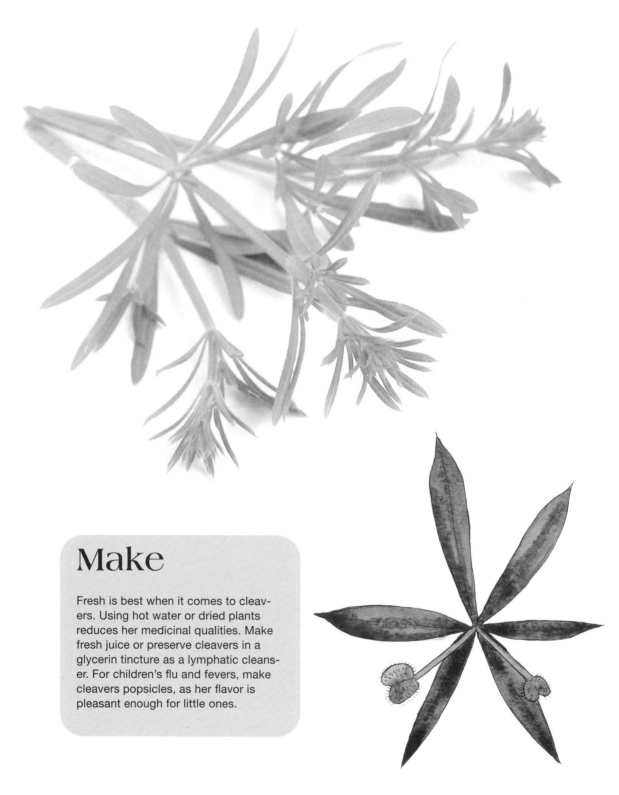

Make

Fresh is best when it comes to cleavers. Using hot water or dried plants reduces her medicinal qualities. Make fresh juice or preserve cleavers in a glycerin tincture as a lymphatic cleanser. For children's flu and fevers, make cleavers popsicles, as her flavor is pleasant enough for little ones.

RED RASPBERRY LEAF

Rubus idaeus

Our Rooted Nations have been revealing their gifts and supporting us with healing remedies since time immortal. Our ancestors only had plants to help for healing. The first recorded use of raspberry's medicine was by the Roman historian Pliny in 37 CE. Her berries gift me with my favorite fruit and her leaf has many healing properties. Raspberry leaf is high in antioxidants and helpful for strengthening the uterine muscles when growing a child in the womb. She is often claimed to help with labor pains, but there are mixed reviews on raspberry leaf's efficacy. It is best to avoid her during the first trimester of pregnancy. She is full of vitamin B, which binds with our hormones and can aid in processing, balancing, and regulating estrogen, testosterone, and progesterone. Raspberry leaf is helpful for diarrhea, menstruation, bronchitis, and sore throats. She contains potassium, calcium, phosphorus, and vitamins A and C.

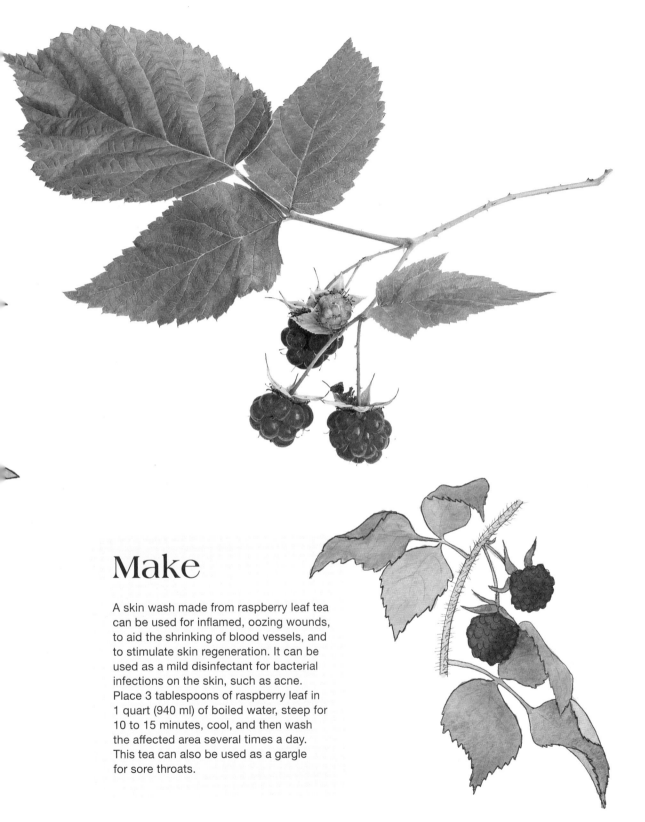

Make

A skin wash made from raspberry leaf tea
can be used for inflamed, oozing wounds,
to aid the shrinking of blood vessels, and
to stimulate skin regeneration. It can be
used as a mild disinfectant for bacterial
infections on the skin, such as acne.
Place 3 tablespoons of raspberry leaf in
1 quart (940 ml) of boiled water, steep for
10 to 15 minutes, cool, and then wash
the affected area several times a day.
This tea can also be used as a gargle
for sore throats.

WILD VIOLET

Viola odorata

In the language of my ancestors, wild violet is known as *waawiye-bagag*, which describes the rounded, butterfly-shaped petals and leaves. Collected in the early spring by the youth and Elders, petals were steeped overnight to create a beautiful bluish purple tea that would be poured over sugared snow as a treat.

This native is one of the first spring flowers that brings us joy as we witness her beauty and the reminder of the warming season soon to bring many gifts of abundance. In my Medicine Wheel garden, we planted her under the wild plum and Saskatoon berry bush. The best variety as an edible plant is *Viola odorata*, as she holds a beautiful scent.

Wild violet is high in vitamin C and beta-carotene. Violas are mucilaginous, anti-inflammatory, and antioxidant and have blood-cleansing properties. Both the flowers and the leaves are edible, and they are delightful when added to wild green salads. She is known to help with childhood eczema and equally helpful for us older folks with dry skin, varicose veins, and even insect bites.

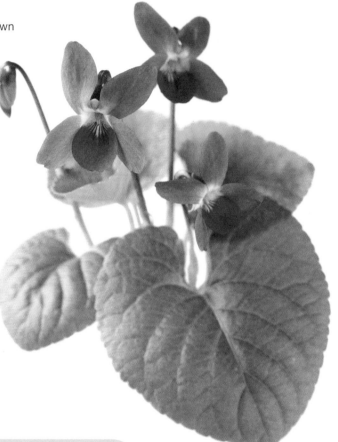

Make

Viola pairs well with sweets like jelly, syrup, cough drops, and candies. Infuse a light white vinegar infusion with violets for 2 weeks and take with honey for a sore throat. Or paint the flower with egg whites and sprinkle with sugar for decorative garnishes. Viola tincture or tea can be taken for her laxative and sedative properties. Since she contains saponins, avoid consuming in large amounts.

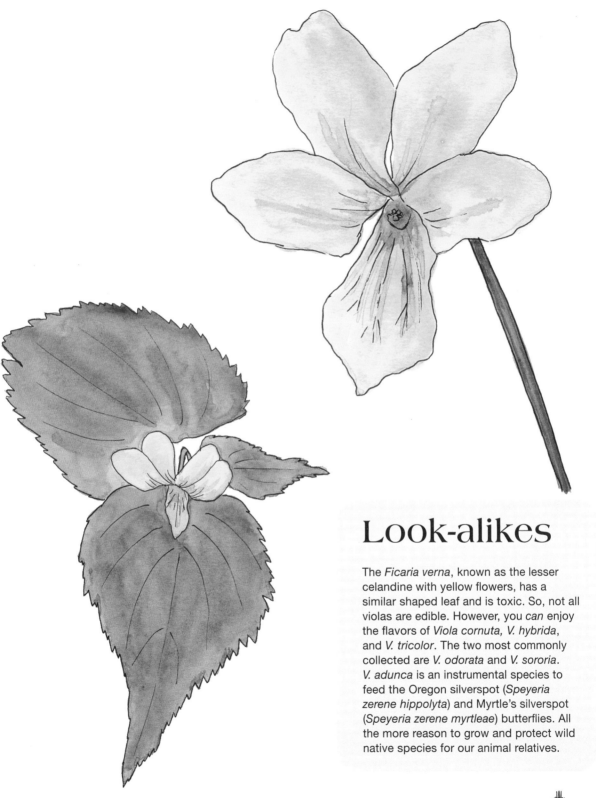

Look-alikes

The *Ficaria verna*, known as the lesser celandine with yellow flowers, has a similar shaped leaf and is toxic. So, not all violas are edible. However, you *can* enjoy the flavors of *Viola cornuta, V. hybrida*, and *V. tricolor*. The two most commonly collected are *V. odorata* and *V. sororia*. *V. adunca* is an instrumental species to feed the Oregon silverspot (*Speyeria zerene hippolyta*) and Myrtle's silverspot (*Speyeria zerene myrtleae*) butterflies. All the more reason to grow and protect wild native species for our animal relatives.

PINE POLLEN

Pinus species

A farmer friend mentioned the amazing attributes offered by pine pollen. He referred to it as plant "Viagra," which I thought he was making up until I came across the book *Pine Pollen: Ancient Medicine for a New Millennium* by Stephen Harrod Buhner. Pine pollen is known as a phytoandrogen, containing many complex compounds to assist our aging population. The plant hormones it contains are similar to testosterone, DHEA, and progesterone in humans. There is much to reclaim from this super supplement and medicine.

Pine pollen is a natraceutical and is known to restore our sleep. Many websites claim their pollen is the best, but my sense is that any pine pollen will be helpful unless you are allergic to it. I understand pine pollen has been used for centuries in Asia in traditional Chinese medicine and for a long period in Europe.

Pine pollen contains over twenty amino acids, eight essential proteins, fifteen different vitamins, thirty minerals, and hundreds of enzymes. This is an active plant steroid. Different species of pine contain different amounts of androgenic hormones. Just like all subspecies, each plant produces more, less, or none at all.

There is a window of time for collecting pine pollen, which is found in ecosystems from sea level to higher elevations. Some foragers cut off the cluster of male cones. I recommend placing a plastic bag over the cluster and then shaking and tapping the branch to help release the pollen. It is a meditative practice, as it takes hours to collect, then sift out bugs and little pieces of plant.

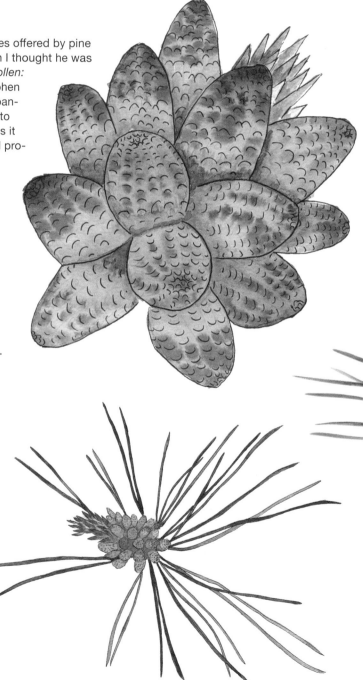

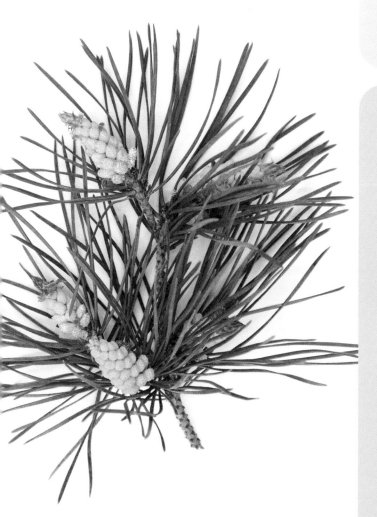

Make

Pine pollen has a hard shell that needs to be frozen or dissolved in 40 percent alcohol. Make a tincture and shake daily for 1 to 2 minutes, storing at room temperature in a dry space. It takes 3 weeks of infusing to access the pollen's goodness. Take a couple of drops under the tongue and put a few drops on the skin to let it absorb into the bloodstream.

Benefits

1. Boosts testosterone to maintain high energy.
2. Prostate regulator via its gibberellins, preventing atrophy or reducing an enlarged prostate.
3. Raises superoxide dismutase levels in the heart, liver, and brain. Protects the body from free radicals by breaking down the oxygen in the cells, preventing damage.
4. Is a potent anti-inflammatory.
5. The brassinolides found in pine pollen and also throughout the plant kingdom assist in germination and new growth of young vegetative tissue. They help detoxify and are also found in wheatgrass and sprouts.
6. Improves fertility, erectile dysfunction, and sperm count. The amino acid arginine is a precursor for nitric oxide, increasing blood flow.
7. Stimulates the immune system via polysaccharides like those found in chaga mushrooms (*Inonotus obliquus*).

COMFREY

Symphytum officinale

The earliest records on comfrey date back to the ancient Greeks, 400 BCE. Named from the Latin word *confervere*, "to join together," "mend," or "heal," traditionally, she was applied to broken bones. She is a powerful cell regenerator, and yet she is widely misunderstood.

Sometimes called "kniit bone," comfrey repairs the bones quickly, as she contains the chemical allantoin. Allantoin acts as an emollient protective film to reduce water loss. Cosmetic companies use synthetic allantoin for products that moisturize, treat acne, and reduce the appearance of fine lines and wrinkles. In her natural form, she is a moisturizer for dry, rough, scaly, and itchy skin, as well as a treatment for scars and skin lesions. Another gift of comfrey leaves is her ability to speed up the decomposing process in your compost pile. Grow comfrey next to the composter, adding leaves when adding more compost to accelerate the process. Traditionally, comfrey leaves longer than 10 inches (25 cm) were collected as food. Today, however, the pyrrolizidine alkaloids are considered toxic to the liver when ingested, according to studies conducted on rats.

Comfrey leaf is fairly large and egg-shaped, with coarse hairs and a wavy edge. She grows in very cool climates and can handle freezing temperatures. Harvest roots in the fall when the plant starts to die back. Collect the smaller rhizomes and replant the central root.

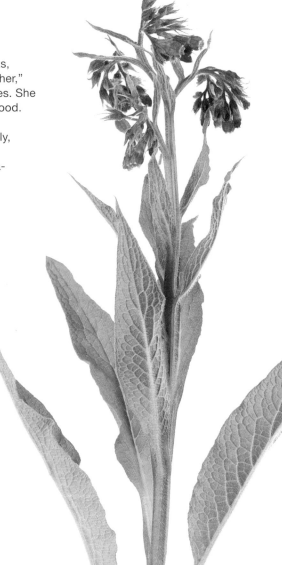

As with all plants of the Rooted Nations, we need to understand their behavior, preferences for growing, and what gifts they offer. Be respectful of the medicines.

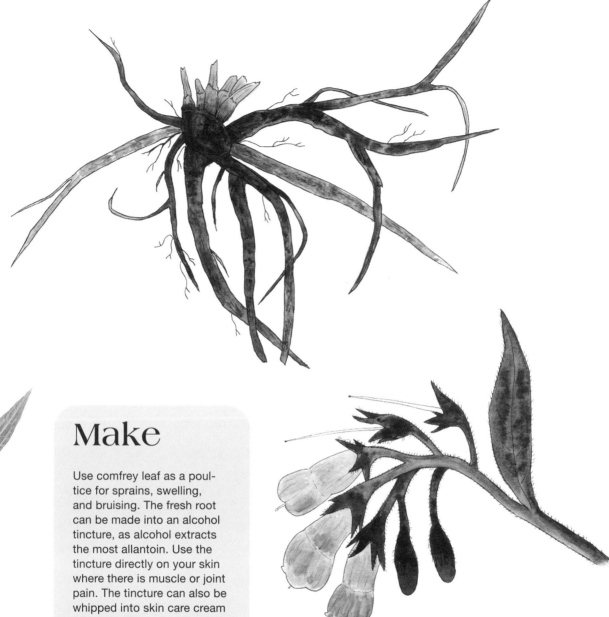

Make

Use comfrey leaf as a poultice for sprains, swelling, and bruising. The fresh root can be made into an alcohol tincture, as alcohol extracts the most allantoin. Use the tincture directly on your skin where there is muscle or joint pain. The tincture can also be whipped into skin care cream recipes for easier application. Use ½ to 1 teaspoon three times daily up to a maximum 3.5 ounces (100 ml) for the week. Do not use for longer than 8 weeks. Do not use on broken skin or open wounds, as the allantoin is so fast acting that the wound could close up the skin before the infection has healed.

Look-alikes

Borage (*Borago officinalis*) is comfrey's kin, but borage flowers are periwinkle in color. Borage is edible and bees love both plants.

HAWTHORN

Crataegus oxyacantha
Crataegus columbiana

Under the canopy of a hawthorn tree blooming during the month of May, I sat with my herb teacher, Don Ollsin, for my very first herb class. Some people may not have chosen to sit below a hawthorn in bloom, as it gives off the unique odor of trimethylamine, a scent associated with sex or when flesh is decaying. This aroma attracts carrion-eating insects. I personally love hawthorn's scent and it's a great biological control in our gardens. She attracts the carnivore insects to eat the herbivore insects, the ones that are eating your greens.

Hawthorn is heart medicine and aids in our ability to digest life. The flowers contain an aromatic lactone that, when swallowed, passes into your digestive tract, then into your bloodstream and flows to open the descending coronary artery in your heart. Various species of hawthorn are found across Turtle Island and many Nations and Tribes ate the stored berries, mixed with fat from marmot, bears, grizzlies, or salmon to make the dried berries more palatable. When eaten in large quantities, some spoke of being susceptible to visions from supernatural beings. The Nlaka'pamux People used the strong wood for digging tools and the thorns for ear piercing and fish hooks. Other Nations burned the leaves, inner bark, and new shoots to paint their faces for winter dances.

In *Grandmother's Secrets: Her Green Guide to Health from Plants*, author Jean Palaiseul wrote that hawthorn is the valerian for the heart made into homeopathic remedies. It reestablishes the equilibrium of the sympathetic and parasympathetic nervous systems. In ancient Greece, she was considered a token of happiness and prosperity for newlyweds. In Rome, a sprig of hawthorn was attached close to newborn babies for protection from sickness and evil spirits.

Hawthorn has an incredibly long history as a heart and digestive medicine. Packed with enzymes, flavonoids, and tannins, the flowers, leaves, and berries offer a tonic for the coronary system. She is also a relaxing nervine, a hypotensive for low blood pressure, and an antioxidant herb.

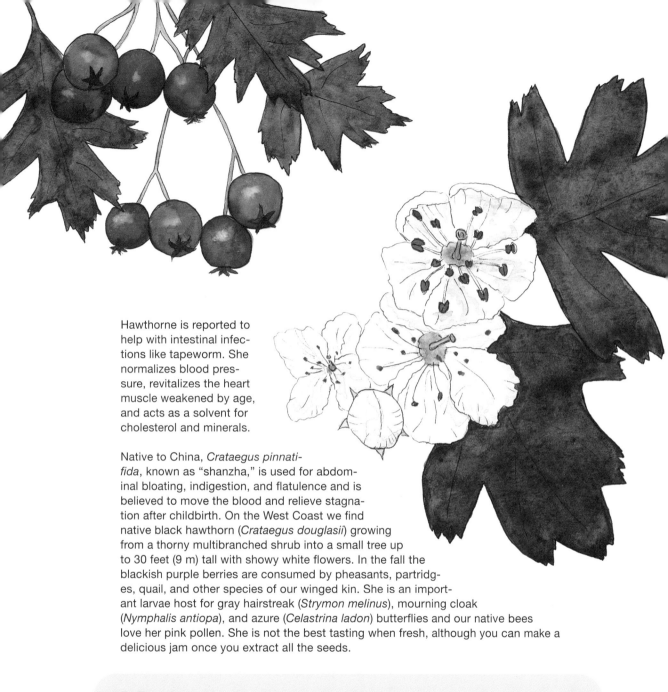

Hawthorne is reported to help with intestinal infections like tapeworm. She normalizes blood pressure, revitalizes the heart muscle weakened by age, and acts as a solvent for cholesterol and minerals.

Native to China, *Crataegus pinnatifida*, known as "shanzha," is used for abdominal bloating, indigestion, and flatulence and is believed to move the blood and relieve stagnation after childbirth. On the West Coast we find native black hawthorn (*Crataegus douglasii*) growing from a thorny multibranched shrub into a small tree up to 30 feet (9 m) tall with showy white flowers. In the fall the blackish purple berries are consumed by pheasants, partridges, quail, and other species of our winged kin. She is an important larvae host for gray hairstreak (*Strymon melinus*), mourning cloak (*Nymphalis antiopa*), and azure (*Celastrina ladon*) butterflies and our native bees love her pink pollen. She is not the best tasting when fresh, although you can make a delicious jam once you extract all the seeds.

Note

It's important to note that hawthorn can increase the effectiveness of heart medications, and as such I advise that you only use her under supervision of a qualified herbalist. Research any contraindications before ingesting pharmaceuticals.

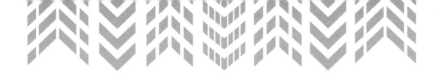

HORSETAIL

Equisetum arvense
Equisetum hyemale
Equisetum telmateia

One of the oldest Rooted Nations on the planet, horsetail is a living fossil dating back to the Devonian period around 350 million years ago. In ancient times she grew as tall as trees. Today, she is a lot shorter. Adapting to the changing climate, field horsetail (*Equisetum arvense*), a fernlike, non-flowering kin, grows only 1 to 2 feet (30 to 61 cm) tall. The giant horsetail (*Equisetum telmateia*) grows up to 6 feet (1.8 m). She is known as souring rush or puzzle plant. The former because the nodes are filled with water you can drink, and the latter because her jointed stems can be easily pulled apart and fit back together like a puzzle.

Horsetail thrives in marshy areas or waterlogged environments, basking in the full sun. She can also flourish in disturbed areas, wastelands, pastures, compacted soils, and even through cracks in the sidewalk. There's much wisdom she can impart to us. She draws minerals from the depths of the earth to the surface, benefiting not just us but also our other relatives.

The giant horsetail was one of the first spring foods along the West Coast that our Indigenous Nations gathered. Gather in the spring when she's a vibrant green, standing at about 12 inches (30 cm) tall, with her whorls (leaves) pointing upward or outward. The fertile shoots can be added to soups or sautés. They are tan in color as they lack chlorophyll. Later in the season, harvest the green stalks of the field horsetail with whorls (leaves) to make mineral medicine. However, the green stalks are not meant to be eaten raw, as they contain thiaminase, an enzyme that destroys vitamin B1. Note that cooking diminishes the enzymes. As she matures, her whorls begin to droop under the weight of silica crystals, which can be irritating to our kidneys. Being mindful of gathering times and paying attention to such details ensures our safety when incorporating her into food or medicine.

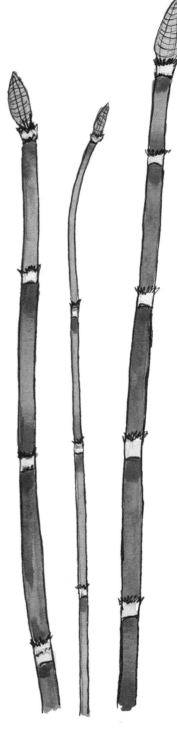

E. hyemale

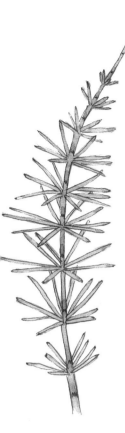

Field horsetail

Horsetail offers many benefits. As a tonic, she fortifies body tissues, and supports the lungs, kidneys, bladder, and sinuses. Her anti-inflammatory qualities, particularly the presence of quercetin, help stabilize mast cells inflamed during allergic reactions. She's been used in treating conditions like bronchitis, tuberculosis, and asthma, often blended with mullein to aid in breaking up dry mucus within the bronchioles and alveoli, the tiny air sacs in the lungs.

Horsetail is rich in silica, which plays a crucial role in building connective tissues such as bones, cartilage, teeth, hair, nails, and arteries. Scouring horsetail (*Equisetum hyemale*) is exceptionally high in silica and can be used to create a tooth powder that helps remineralize our teeth. It's essential to ensure that the harvesting site is free from agricultural and industrial waste, such as inorganic nitrogen, as these contaminants can accumulate in horsetail. Additionally, it's advisable to consult with your health practitioner before using horsetail, as it may interact with certain medications.

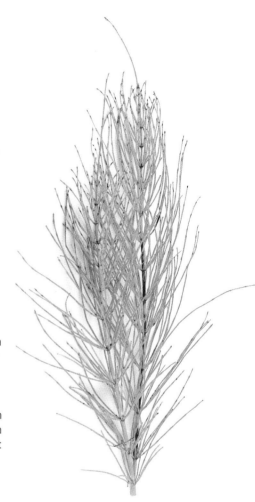

Make

Dry horsetail, blend, and put it in capsules for menopausal hair loss and to strengthen the kidneys. Blend with other mineral-rich herbs like red clover, chickweed, peppermint, stinging nettles, and yarrow. Infuse them into cider vinegars for added minerals. Make horsetail tea to help alleviate the burning sensation caused by acute kidney tract infections. Drink it for 1 month and then take a week off. The recommended dose is ½ to 1 teaspoon dried horsetail in 1 cup (240 ml) of boiling water, simmered for 5 minutes, or infused for 30 minutes in cold water. Consume 2 to 3 cups (480 to 720 ml) daily.

Create a tooth powder by combining ¼ cup bentonite clay, 2 teaspoons aluminum-free baking soda (omit if you have braces), ½ teaspoon activated charcoal (optional), 10 to 20 drops peppermint essential oil (or spearmint, clove, or tea tree), and 2 teaspoons dried horsetail. Adjust the ingredients to your preference and experiment by adding cinnamon, ground cloves, stevia, or ground mint. Store the mixture in a glass jar. Wet your toothbrush and dip the bristles in the powder before brushing.

PAPER BIRCH

Betula papyrifera

Grandfather Birch is one of the sacred trees for the Anishinaabe People, spoken as *wiigwaasaatig*, and for the Cree People, spoken as *waskway*. There will be variation from region to region with spelling and pronunciation. A prevalent tree within the Great Lakes area and spiritually connected to the Indigenous People, paper birch offers many teachings and gifts. Made into baskets, the birch bark formed the outside of the canoe, is helpful as a fire starter, roof covering, food, and medicine. She is found growing in the circumboreal areas of Europe, Asia, and Russia. The Russian people too have a deep relationship with paper birch.

Gathered from the larger paper birch, as it contains more sugars and starches, the inner bark is edible for those times when food was scarce. The inner bark can be sliced into strips and cooked like spaghetti noodles or dried and crushed to be used as flour. Collect the bark at any time of year, although the spring is best, as the sap is rising. Take care to not cut too deep and girdle or damage the tree. Her cut will heal, but it will not grow back white. Paper birch bark contains large amounts of the triterpene betulin and small amounts of betulinic acid, which may be helpful for various cancers, like skin, brain, and ovarian. Her bark has been dried and powdered to use for rashes and baby's bums.

The sap water is even sweeter than the inner bark. Tap birch trees in the early spring before the leaves have emerged. Collect the young leaves in spring as the leaves unfurl to use fresh or dried in tinctures or an infusion for the urinary system. Paper birch is antirheumatic, astringent, and lithontriptic (has the ability to dissolve stones in the bladder or kidneys). Grandfather Birch is a tonic, diuretic, anti-inflammatory, antiseptic, and considered anticancer.

> "Man esteems himself happy, when that which is his food is also his medicine."
> —Alma Hutchens, *Indian Herbalogy of North America*

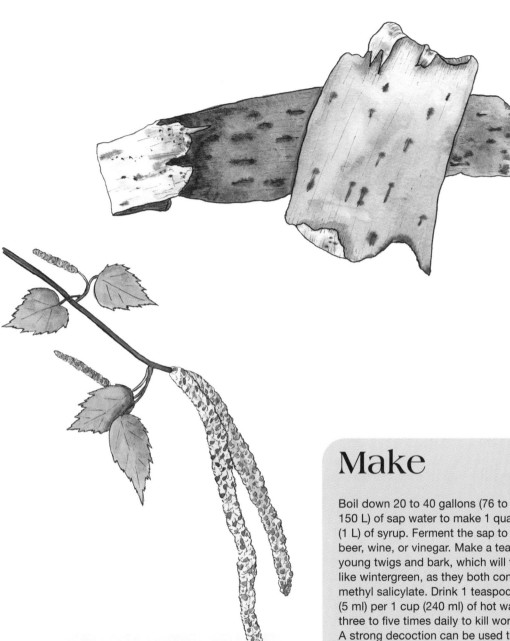

Make

Boil down 20 to 40 gallons (76 to 150 L) of sap water to make 1 quart (1 L) of syrup. Ferment the sap to make beer, wine, or vinegar. Make a tea with young twigs and bark, which will taste like wintergreen, as they both contain methyl salicylate. Drink 1 teaspoon (5 ml) per 1 cup (240 ml) of hot water three to five times daily to kill worms. A strong decoction can be used to treat eczema externally. A plant-derived substance made from the paper birch bark is the sugar substitute xylitol, reported to help with cavities, although be mindful that xylitol is poisonous to our pets.

Musings

We can also find chaga mushrooms (*Inonotus obliquus*) growing on the bark. Make a tonic with chaga to cleanse the blood.

NODDING ONION, WILD LEEK, AND WILD GARLIC

Allium cernuum
Allium tricoccum
Allium ursinum

In the book *Florilegio Medicinal*, published in 1711, author Juan de Esteyneffer compiled a list of common herbal medicines found in Europe and among Native People. Allium appeared most frequently for her medicinal properties to treat headaches, earaches, ulcers, wounds, coughs, and burns. She is a helpful cold remedy, eases sore throats, is a febrifuge to reduce fevers, and aids the gastrointestinal tract, kidneys, and liver. Western science confirms her antibacterial, antifungal, and antiviral properties. The high sulfur and flavonoid content helps prevent disease and enhances our health.

There are many species of allium growing across Turtle Island. Three you might consider growing in your garden are nodding onion, wild leek, and wild garlic. Nodding onion, which blooms May to July, is a perennial with long, thin, flat basal leaves. She has pink and white bulbs growing in clusters that produce a strong flower stalk. Her pink flower umbels hang downward, or "nod." Children love to snack on her pungent, spicy, oniony leaf. Known as *ajo-cebolla* in Spanish, and in Latin as *unio*, meaning "onion," she likes dry open woods, edges of large trees, exposed grassy areas, borders along lawns, and rocky crevices or rock gardens. Collect her bulbs anytime other than when flowering. Dig up the larger bulbs and leave the smaller ones for next year's crop. The leaf, bulb, and flowers are edible. If you are sensitive to sulfides, which inhibit fungal and bacterial growth, avoid them or only eat a few at a time. Her leaf is sweetest in the spring, when it contains the highest amounts of vitamins A, B, and C, phosphorus, calcium, magnesium, sulfur, sodium, iron, and potassium.

Wild leek (*Allium tricoccum*) is also known as spring onion or ramps. We find her growing in calcium-rich, slightly acidic soil, in moist areas like floodplains and drainages on northern slopes. She is an indicator plant of community, as we find her under the canopy of sugar maple (*Acer saccharum*) and blue cohosh (*Caulophyllum thalictroides*). On floodplains, wild leek grows with Jack-in-the-pulpit (*Arisaema triphyllum*), mayapple (*Podophyllum peltatum*), and bitternut hickory (*Carya cordiformis*). Wild turkeys love to eat the seeds.

Wild garlic

 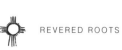

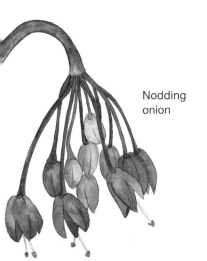

Nodding onion

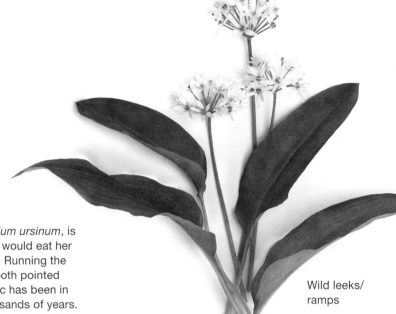

Wild leeks/ramps

Wild garlic's Latin name, *Allium ursinum*, is named for bears (*Ursi*), who would eat her pungent, spear-shaped leaf. Running the length of her long, thin, smooth pointed leaf are little lines. Wild garlic has been in relationship with us for thousands of years. We find accounts to support her use with the Egyptians, Greeks, and Vikings. Sadly, with the loss of habitat and development, there is less wild garlic growing. In 1995, the province of Quebec enacted section 16 of the Threatened and Vulnerable Species Act, banning the harvesting of wild garlic for commercial sale. This created increased demand for and made smuggling common practice. She can be collected for personal use, up to fifty bulbs per person, per year. Do not harvest from the thirty-nine protected parks.

Look-alikes

● Death camus (*Toxicoscordion venenosum*) with her white flower can be mistaken for nodding onion. One important way to identify it is by rubbing the leaf and smelling. Does it smell like onion? If it does not, then it is not nodding onion.

● Lily of the valley (*Convallaria majalis*) and *Arum maculatum*, known as Adam and Eve or cuckoo plant, can be mistaken for wild garlic.

Make

● Nodding onion can be eaten raw or cooked. Pickle, boil, sauté, and add to soups for a sweet onion flavor. Chop the leaves and infuse with chamomile in cold water overnight to make a fungicide spray for your plants.

● Collect a few leaves and add to your sandwiches. Pickle the flower heads. When cooked, a more delicate, sweeter flavor emerges.

Musings

Grow our More-Than-Human-Kin in guilds/communities to support each other. Nodding onions like to be with roses, carrots, beets, and chamomile.

SORRELS

Rumex acetosella
Oxalis oregana
Oxalis acetosella

Common sorrel, also known as sheep sorrel (*Rumex acetosella*), is great for salads, soups, stews, and puddings as she has a tangy lemon flavor that the children love. Sheep sorrel's root contains fat-soluble vitamin A for skin, vision, and reproductive health, along with vitamin C and antioxidants to help the body resist infections. She also contains B complex, vitamins K and E, calcium, magnesium, sulfur, zinc, silicon, manganese, iodine, potassium, beta-carotene, and chlorophyll, plus citric, tannic, oxalic, and tartaric acids.

Redwood sorrel (*Oxalis oregana*) is a native low-growing herbaceous ground cover. She loves the moist shaded space found along the West Coast. Her heart-shaped, trifoliate clover leaf is a tasty, tangy bite to snack on. A native tuber, *Oxalis tuberosa*, was a prominent food crop prior to the Spanish arriving in the Andes. The roots were higher in protein, antioxidants, amino acids, and fiber than potatoes and more nutritious than spinach. Medicinally, she has been used for scurvy, fevers, urinary tract infections, canker sores, nausea, and sore throats. An introduced species, *Oxalis pes-caprae*, indigenous to South Africa, acts as a mordant for dying cellulose and protein fibers for her yellowish orange color.

Wood sorrel (*Oxalis acetosella*), like the other sorrels, has a lemony citrus, green apple flavor. An early spring green found in many places worldwide, she is easy to include in your recipes. All parts are edible. Her flowers attract bees, ants, and butterflies.

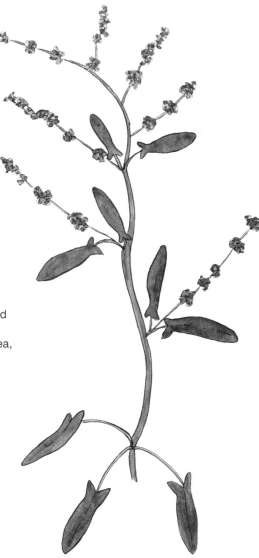

Common sorrel

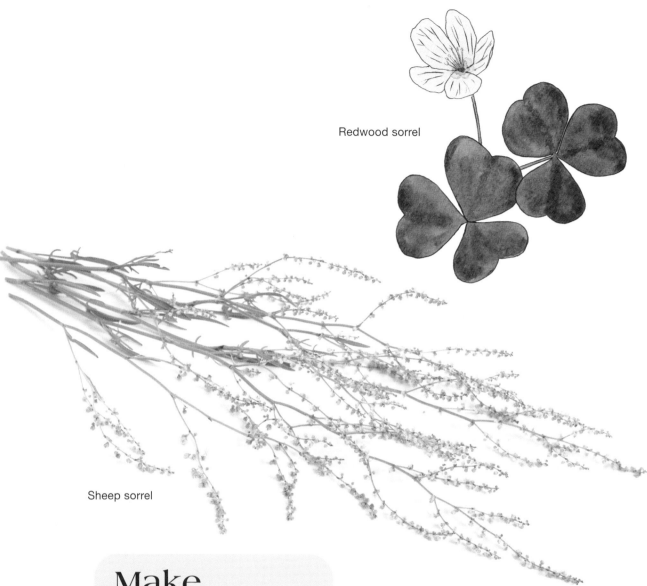

Redwood sorrel

Sheep sorrel

Make

Some of my favorite ways to use sorrel are in a sour tart made with cream and topped with raspberries. Sorrel can also be used in a savory quiche, in a simple sugar syrup for flavoring drinks, in a tea to gargle with for mouth ulcers, or in an alcohol tincture taken for constipation and chronic pain.

Note

Do not consume in large quantities as the oxalic acid inhibits the absorption of calcium. Avoid if you have gout, rheumatism, or kidney stones or are pregnant.

PURPLE DEAD NETTLE AND HENBIT

Lamium purpureum
Lamium amplexicaule

Purple dead nettle (*Lamium purpureum*) is a harbinger of spring. She is part of the mint family, as is her relative, henbit (*Lamium amplexicaule*). The leaves are green, turning more purple, pink, or red toward the top of the plant; however, the color may indicate lack of nutrients in the soil. It's best to gather her leaves before the flower blooms to avoid the formation of cystolith crystals. The seed has a little appendage called an elaiosome, which is a little clear, white speck and is a nutritious food for ants. Ants are known to disperse seeds from trilliums, bloodroot (*Sanguinaria canadensis*), wild ginger, Pacific bleeding heart (*Dicentra formosa*), and trout lily (*Erythronium americanum*). Bumblebees and native bees are grateful for the nectar and pollen provided by purple dead nettle.

Purple dead nettle, like so many other plants, contains many different chemical compounds that offer a range of health benefits, including use as an astringent, diuretic, diaphoretic, purgative, anti-inflammatory, antibacterial, and antifungal. She also is styptic like yarrow and frog's leaf (plantain). Purple dead nettle has been used to treat scurvy, as she is full of vitamin C, iron, and potassium. Both purple dead nettle and henbit are great foods for chickens, rabbits, and ducks. Avoid dead nettle, henbit, and creeping Charlie when pregnant or breastfeeding. In general, it is best to consume her in smaller quantities.

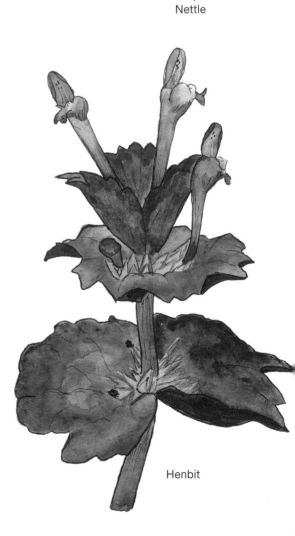

Purple Dead Nettle

Henbit

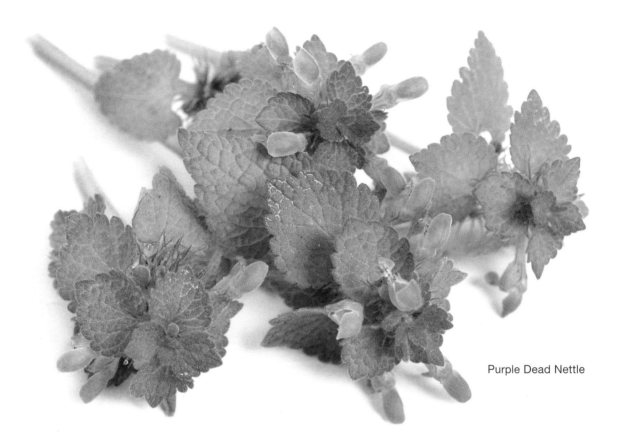

Purple Dead Nettle

Make

Blend purple dead nettle and henbit with other wild greens to make pesto or green sauces. Add a lot of garlic. Steep for tea or prepare an alcohol tincture for allergies. Make a poultice with fresh or powdered purple dead nettle to stop a wound from bleeding.

Look-alikes

Henbit is another relative of the mint family. She has scalloped leaves attaching around the stem (known as sessile), with tubular pink flowers and fine hairs on the hood. The good news is both plants are edible. Creeping Charlie, or ground ivy (*Glechoma hederacea*), is another edible and medicine.

Purple dead nettle has been known to harbor tomato spotted wilt virus.

YARROW

Achillea millefolium

Our interconnection with yarrow has a long history. We find her growing all around the circumference of the globe, inviting many cultures to be engaged and in relationship with her. The Aleut and Unangan Peoples around Alaska rolled the leaves and placed them over cuts. She contains the alkaloid achilleine, which facilitates coagulation, closing the wound rapidly. Yarrow fresh or dried flowers and leaves are great to use for nosebleeds, stopping them almost immediately. Yarrow is a native aromatic perennial, growing up to 2 feet (61 cm) tall with a flat, round cluster of little flowers. I recommend you taste her, as she offers her seasonal bitter leaves to activate our stagnant digestion.

As a vulnerary (the ability to heal wounds), yarrow was used by the Menominee of the northeastern United States. Known as the "wild rice people," they rubbed the fresh tops on eczema sores and used the leaves as poultices for children's rashes. The Zuni of New Mexico ground up the entire plant, mixed it with cold water, and applied it on burns. The Klallam People of the Olympic Peninsula in Washington State chewed the leaves to put on sores. The Chippewa from the United States and Canada made a decoction to apply externally for skin eruptions. The Chippewa also sprinkled dried leaves on hot stones to inhale the fumes for headaches. The Squaxin, descendants of several Lushootseed clans in western Washington, crushed the flowers for skin sores. For rheumatism, the Quinault People on the Pacific Coast of Washington laid the boiled leaves on rheumatic limbs and used it to reduce fevers. They made teas as eyewashes and boiled the root for a tonic and to treat tuberculosis. The Winnebago, whose historical territories include Wisconsin, Minnesota, Iowa, and Illinois, used yarrow in baths for swelling as she increases circulation and cardiovascular activity.

Yarrow is a diaphoretic, which helps reduce a high fever through increased sweating. For the relief of diarrhea, the Snohomish People of the Lushootseed-speaking Tribe in the Puget Sound region of Washington State, along with the Skagit People, used yarrow for diarrhea. The Chehalis of Washington State boiled the leaves to stop the flow of blood found in diarrhea. The Cowlitz Tribe from Washington State used yarrow for hair care. She promotes healthy hair growth,

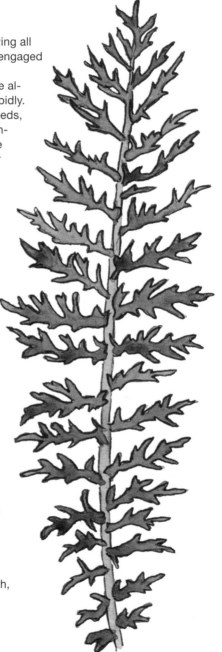

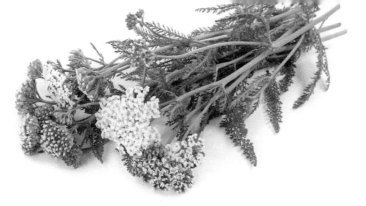

reduces inflammation on the scalp, removes buildup of shampoos, and strengthens the hair shaft. The Klallam People in the Olympic Peninsula mixed it with wild cherry bark for colds and flus. In Kenai, Alaska, the Dena'ina Athabaskan People boiled the plant in water for steaming. The Cheyenne People of the Great Plains drank infusions for coughs, colds, and nausea. The Mi'kmaq from the Atlantic provinces of Canada boiled the plant in milk for 1 hour to cure colds.

Yarrow attracts predators and parasitic insects to prey upon herbivores and help balance your garden ecosystem. She is also an amazing pollinator plant. Butterflies love her nectar and she is a larval host plant for moths and beetles. She is one of the prettiest perennials for cut flower arrangements. By and large, yarrow offers many gifts for us to rediscover.

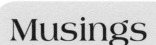

Look-alikes

Fool's parsley (*Aethusa cynapium*) and poison hemlock (*Conium maculatum*) can be confused for yarrow.

Make

Brew a strong tea with the leaves for a soothing footbath.

Musings

One of the most powerful ways we can take plant medicines into the body is through footbaths and bathing. Our feet have over 72,000 nerve endings and six main meridians for acupuncture. Traditional Chinese medicine teaches us that the body is a tree. Our head is the branches, the body is the trunk, and the feet are the roots. To treat illnesses, we water the roots.

Check out https://native-land.ca to discover whose traditional lands you are living on.

LAMB'S QUARTER

Chenopodium album

One of the top five books in my emergency bag is Katrina Blair's book, *The Wild Wisdom of Weeds: 13 Essential Plants for Human Survival*. She writes of the thirteen wild botanicals dispersed around the world that are successfully resilient though their ability to thrive in the most adverse environments. They thrive in diverse conditions, break through compacted soil, create shade, bring minerals from the deep earth, and lay down their leaves to replenish our depleted soils. Wild weeds grow when we expose Mother Earth. They are known as "people plants," growing around us in everyday spaces. They are considered a part of a successional regenerative process to bring equilibrium to unbalance ecosystems.

Lamb's quarter, also known as goosefoot or pigweed, is one of these top thirteen wild weeds. *Chenopodium* is Greek for "goosefoot" and *album* is Latin for "white." Her leaves are covered with a fine silvery, waxy film that helps hold moisture, like a succulent. Full of minerals, lamb's quarter is a self-seeding branching annual, growing 3 to 5 feet (1 to 1.5 m) tall. Her stem is variegated and lined, with alternating leaves that are green on the top and triangular, diamond, or goose-shaped with coarsely soft-toothed edges. The smaller leaves at the top of the herb are more arrow-shaped. Non-showy inflorescences are spiked with tight whitish, green, or yellow flowers at the terminal ends. This is followed by a thin pericarp wall with a minuscule kidney-shaped seed head that is either black, brown, or reddish, producing upwards of 75,000 seeds. The seeds appear in late summer. Roll her leaves between your fingers to smell her spinach-like aroma.

Within the genus there are 170 species, all of which are edible. Lamb's quarter is our "wild spinach." Harvest the tops and eat them fresh in small amounts. She contains oxalate acid, which you can neutralize by adding lemon. Oxalic acid binds with minerals, decreasing mineral uptake and increasing the formation of kidney stones. When trying a new herb, it's good practice to eat one wild botanical at a time so you know whether there are any reactions. Let your tongue be your guide, and if the flavor is too strong, use less or not at all.

Dry the leaves, grind them into a powder, and make vitamin supplement capsules. Lamb's quarter, amaranth, and purslane are considered the three most nutritious wild weeds available. Lamb's quarter is full of vitamins A, B1, and B2, as well as protein and fiber. Reconstitute the dried powder by mixing it with water to make tortillas. The leaves are on the salty side, making her a good choice for a seasoning mix. When the leaves are older you may experience a burning sensation in your throat.

Make

Lamb's quarter seeds make highly nutritious sprouted greens. Use dried fruit, sunflower seeds, bee pollen, and 1 tablespoon of dried leaf to make energy bars. Leave the seeds for winter food for our winged relatives. Juice the leaves, which are full of chlorophyll and will help chelate and detoxify toxins. Make a tea for an astringent mouthwash. Blanching and freezing is another way to preserve the leaves for the winter. Shampoo soap can be made with her root. Root tea is cleansing, works as a laxative, and can be made into a poultice for pain, swelling, or rheumatism. Teas are helpful for diarrhea, skin ailments, stomachaches, and loss of appetite.

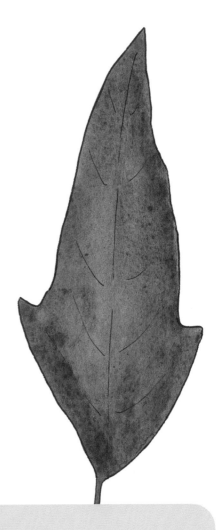

I found Daniel Shelton Robinson's thesis from the University of Tennessee, who researched one of our native species of *Chenopodium berlandieri*. It appears she is one of our first domesticated relationships dating back to the end of the Ice Age around ten thousand years ago. He researched about the Eastern Agricultural Complex that included a selection of various species prior to the domestication of corn (*Zea mays*): squash (*Cucurbita pepo*), goosefoot (*Chenopodium berlandieri*), erect knotweed (*Polygonum erectum*), maygrass (*Phalaris caroliniana*), marsh elder (*Iva annua*), and sunflower (*Helianthus annuus*). These plants contain oily or starchy seeds and edible leafy matter for sustenance. The evidence of the domestication of *Chenopodium berlandieri* is an interesting find, as seeds were found in the Newt Kash and Cloudsplitter rock shelters in eastern Kentucky, leading to his hypothesis: Food is medicine.

continued on next page

Look-alikes

Several plants from the *Solanum* (night-shade) genus, including *Solanum nigrum, S. villosum, S. physalifolium*, and *S. sarrachoides*, have been mistaken for lamb's quarter. Another look-alike is nettle-leaf goosefoot (*Chenopodiastrum murale*).

Musings

Pungent, bitter tastes have always been considered medicine. It is a privilege to grow our wild foods outside our doors, offered from Mother Earth as they reach toward the sky.

Make

Use as a flavoring ingredient when cooking beans. The two phytochemical compounds, geraniol and safrole, are found in the leaf and stem. These antibacterial agents allow the beans to remain edible for a longer time before any bacteria sets in, inhibiting spoilage before they can be finished being consumed. Prepare with 1 tablespoon of dried lamb's quarter for every ½ cup (125 g) of dried beans.

Note

Some folks have reported allergies to her pollen.

HERB ROBERT

Geranium robertianum

Found worldwide in Europe, China, Japan, Africa, and North and South America, herb robert has long been used in folklore medicine. The National Library of Medicine published an article in 2023 on *Geranium robertianum*, writing that she is "a valuable medicinal for those hard to heal wounds." The study acknowledges her anticancer potential for pharyngeal and colon cancers, an antiviral against herpes virus type 1, and an antibacterial for Candida fungi. The research cited forty-two articles on herb robert.

Flowering from May to October, she sports little pinkish mauve flowers that grow on a small annual up to 15 inches (38 cm) tall. She is easy to identify, with long, red stems with tiny hairs. Herb robert has a sharp, distinctive, "foxy" smell. She can grow out of cracks in the sidewalk but is easy to pull out of Mother Earth. In Montenegro, her aerial parts are used for diarrhea, stomach inflammation, and diseases of the urinary system. Traditionally, she was carried to bring good luck and fertility.

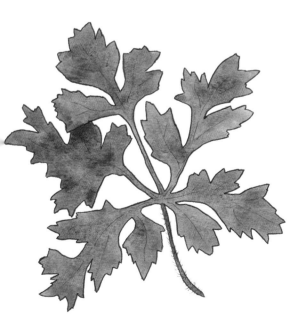

Musings

Could this be your medicine growing around you?

Make

Herb robert is considered a spicy, potable herb to eat. Collect the leaf to make a tea and use it as a gargle for sore throats, toothaches, and mouth ulcers or as a brown dye. Rub fresh leaves on your skin to repel mosquitoes.

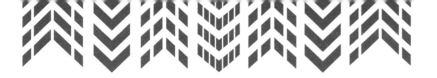

PURSLANE

Portulaca oleracea

Purslane shows up as a red-stemmed ground cover, growing close to Mother Earth, reaching out, spreading like a spiderweb. As she grows outward, protecting the soil, she becomes a shade corridor for insects. Stabilizing ground moisture, purslane creates a humid microclimate for nearby neighboring Kin. Her deep taproot reaches down through hard compacted soil, bringing up moisture and nutrients for her community of More-Than-Human-Kin. Corn roots have been found to follow purslane roots through denser soil that corn would not be able to penetrate on her own (this is known in Western science as ecological facilitation). Deposits of purslane were found at Crawford Lake, Ontario, dating back to 1430 CE. She is enjoyed by many cultures in Europe, the Middle East, and Mexico. The Aborigines in Australia used the seeds to make seed cakes also known as bush bread.

Sometimes known as portulaca, she is mucilaginous in her texture, with a sour, salty, lemony flavor. Purslane is filled with omega-3s, a super nutrient for our brains that also lowers blood pressure. Just 3.5 ounces (100 g) equals 300 to 400 mg of omega-3. She contains two types of betalains: red betacyanins, a potent antioxidant and a yellow betaxanthins, an antimutagen. She mines the deep minerals and provides potassium, protein, magnesium, iron, calcium, pectin, and vitamins A, B6, C, and E.

During the photosynthesis process, purslane switches to the crassulacean acid metabolism, where at night she traps carbon dioxide and converts it to malic acid. In the daytime the malic acid is converted to glucose. This means that by collecting her in the early morning, her leaves have ten times more malic acid and will taste tangier, while in the afternoon she will taste less tangy.

Medicinally, purslane helps with insect bites, diarrhea, hemorrhoids, post-partum bleeding, intestinal bleeding, arthritis, and inflammation. In Traditional Chinese Medicine, she is prescribed for respiratory and circulatory ailments. Studies have shown that she removes bisphenol A, an endocrine-disrupting hormone. Purslane contains mutagenic properties, where she helps cells from mutating. Do not use when pregnant or if you have weak digestion.

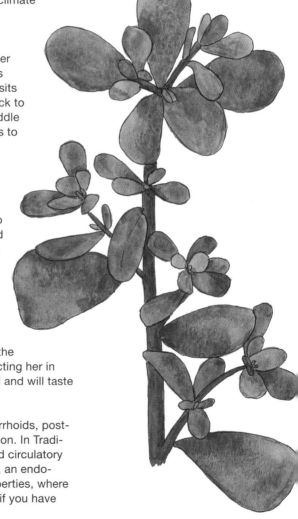

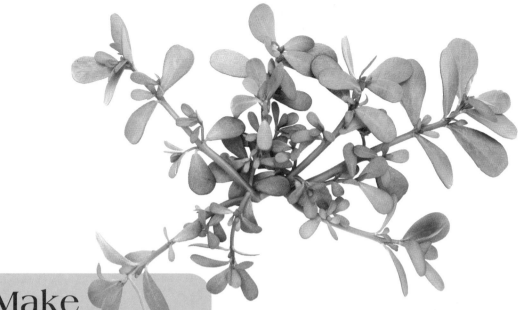

Make

Purslane is best eaten fresh. To store, wrap in a moist paper towel, wrap in plastic, and store in the fridge. You can substitute it for spinach, use it in pesto (use less oil), pickle it, or add it as a thickener for soups and stews. For a classic Crete recipe, combine 2½ cups (600 g) strained thick yogurt, 1 cup (30 g) coarsely chopped purslane, 1 cup (40 g) coarsely chopped romaine lettuce, ¼ cup (60 ml) olive oil, 3½ tablespoons (52 ml) red wine vinegar, 2 tablespoons (16 g) capers, and 1 teaspoon minced garlic.

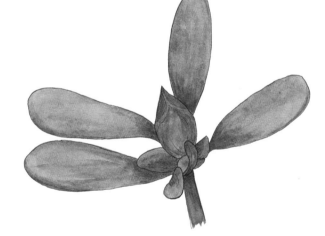

Notes

Enjoy the freshness and unique flavors of our wild foods. Purslane is prolific in her seed production, producing up to 200,000 per year. Her seeds are variable for up to forty years as long as the seeds are not more than ½ inch (1.3 cm) below the soil.

Morning is a good time to gather purslane just after the dew has dried and before the day has become too hot. Remember, ask permission, and leave an offering. Collect only what you need; this way you won't feel overwhelmed and nothing will go to waste. Thank you, Creator, for providing us with all that we need.

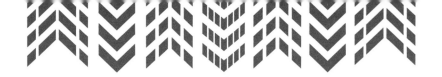

FIREWEED

Chamaenerion angustifolium

Fireweed is an important contributor to Indigenous People living around the circumference of our planet. The delicate fluff of silk from the seed pod was used for fiber in weaving and for padding by many Nations. A high-ranking member of various Nations within British Columbia would have grown a personal patch of fireweed. Known as a "pioneer," fireweed regenerates the soil and fosters an environment that sustains a strong, diverse plant community. She is the first one to appear after a forest fire, after a volcanic eruption, at logging sites, or in other disturbed areas.

Prior to the arrival of tea (*Camellia sinensis*) from China, fireweed leaf was predominately drunk as our native tea. The tea leaf helps the small intestine with beneficial bacteria to assist with nutrient absorption and for waste to move out of our bodies. She acts as a gentle but effective anti-inflammatory. The tannins work as an astringent, toning the colon and slowing the amount of water being reabsorbed back into the body. For the gut, she is a mild laxative and antifungal for Candida over-growth in the intestines.

In the Indigenous communities along the Pacific Coast, this was one of the first vegetable foods of spring, along with salmonberry and thimbleberry shoots. Gather when young, when the leaves are growing upward, by snapping the shoot off at the base. Scoop out the inner pith to eat. The leaf can be pinched off and prepared like spinach. It's best to collect the leaves before they become too fibrous with age. For a tea rich with vitamin A, collect the leaf just before she blooms at the height of the summer solstice. Once the leaf is dried, she releases her berry and citrus tones. Fireweed is helpful when recovering from food poisoning and soothes irritable bowel syndrome.

Fireweed is classified in the Onagraceae (evening primrose) family and is my all-time favorite flower. She grows up to 7 feet (2.1 m) tall, with brilliant pink, magenta, rose, or purple flowers. *Angustifolium*, Latin for "narrow leaf," carries this unique feature where the leaf veins are circular where they don't terminate at the edges, which makes for easy identification. Producing up to 80,000 seeds on a little tuft of silk hairs for wind dispersal, traveling great distances, she reproduces both by seeds and through rhizomes. Be mindful that her root system can take over the garden. You can also collect her roots, which are edible raw or steamed. They are high in vitamins A and C and helpful for the prostate gland.

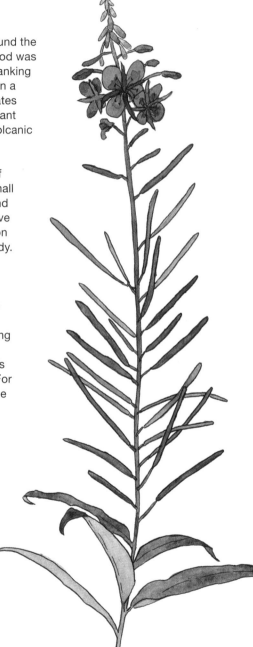

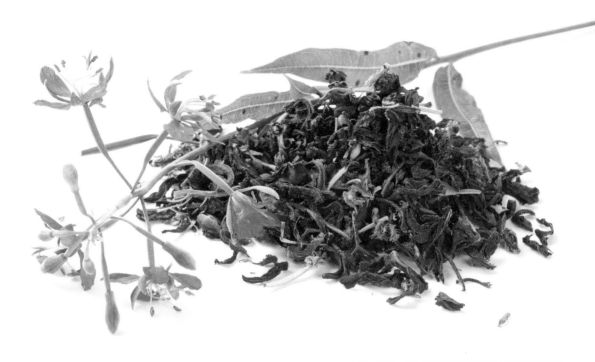

Musings

As a vital pollinator plant, fireweed flowers produce plentiful nectar for the bees who gift us with a rich, spicy, flavorful honey.

Make

Steep tea with 1 tablespoon dried leaves in 1 cup (240 ml) boiling water for 15 minutes and drink three times daily. Make a strong decoction with the flowers and use it to make fireweed jelly. Infuse the flowers and leaves in oil for a healing skin salve for burns and skin abrasions. I apply infused fireweed flower facial oil as my moisturizer.

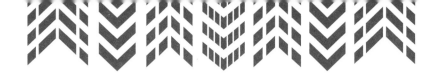

OXEYE DAISY

Leucanthemum vulgare

A member of the Asteraceae family, oxeye daisy in ancient times was dedicated to Diana, the goddess of the moon, and later dedicated to Mary Magdalene, symbolizing patience. She is referred to as moon daisy because she does not close up during the night like her cousins, dandelion and other daisies.

Oxeye daisy is an import from Europe and found mostly in waste areas. She is both an indicator of poor soil conditions, remediating and remineralizing the upper level of our soil. The Latin name, *Leucanthemum*, refers to "white flower." Shasta daisy (*Leucanthemum* x *superbum*), a hybridized flower, grows larger with glossy, thicker succulent leaves and a larger flower head and is bred to adorn flower garden beds.

Oxeye daisy's solitary, white daisy flower stands up to 3 feet (91 cm) tall and is attractive to pollinators. All her aerial parts are edible and one of the most unique wild greens I have ever tasted. The edible parts have been described as spicy, bitter, nutty, strangely sweet, and green. Nonetheless, her greens can be added to casseroles, salads, sandwiches, wraps, tacos, and spring rolls. Pickle her flowers in leftover pickle brine or pickle the flower buds like capers. Oxeye daisy seeds are full of fiber, protein, and fats, plus the flavonoids glutamine and quercetin. She holds medicinal qualities for bronchitis, colds, fevers, sore throats, loss of appetite, cramps, whooping cough, asthma, and nervousness.

Note

Oxeye daisy is poisonous to dogs due to her sesquiterpene lactones.

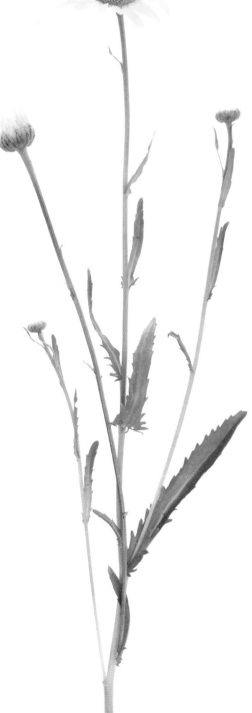

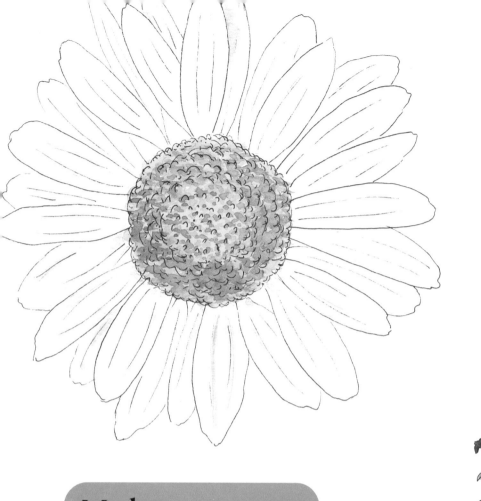

Make

Steep her flowers for tea to help calm the nervous system. Simmer the leaf and stalk and sweeten it with honey for chronic coughs and night sweats. Infuse in oil to make a balm for sore muscles and wounds.

Look-alikes

Oxeye daisy is sometimes confused with stinking mayweed (*Anthemis cotula*), prairie fleabane (*Erigeron strigosus*), or false chamomile (*Tripleurospermum inodorum*).

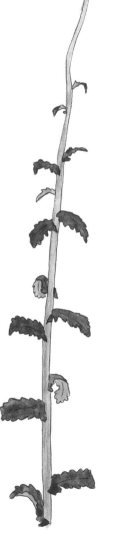

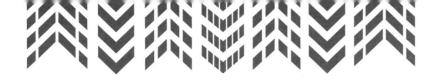

OATSTRAW

Avena sativa

A descendant of *Avena sterilis* and a cross between wheat and barley, our present-day oatstraw is an herbal favorite. She has a long history dating back to the Fertile Crescent along the Tigris and Euphrates Rivers. Hildegard of Bingen, a nun and herbalist born in 1098, referred to oatstraw as one of her top five "happiness" herbs. In the seventeenth century, oatstraw was grown to feed the draft horses on family farms. Today, she is cultivated worldwide for cattle and horse feed, commercial cosmetics, and food. Her nutritive, restorative properties help us with burnout, cold, depleted energy, and chronic tiredness.

A common cereal grain, oatstraw gives us fortitude as a formidable food source. My Scottish ancestors started the trend of eating oats for breakfast, as they are full of calcium, iron, manganese, magnesium, zinc, and vitamins A, B, C, E, and K. Oatstraw's steroidal saponins, polysaccharides, and lignins nourish the pancreas, adrenals, and liver. By reducing inflammation, she expands the arteries in the brain, bringing more blood, reviving brain function, and modulating our hormones to restore our moods. As a probiotic starch, she stabilizes our blood sugars, strengthens our bones and teeth, and lowers cholesterol. Oatstraw has no known drug interactions. Use a water infusion method to capture her water-soluble constituents instead of an alcohol tincture.

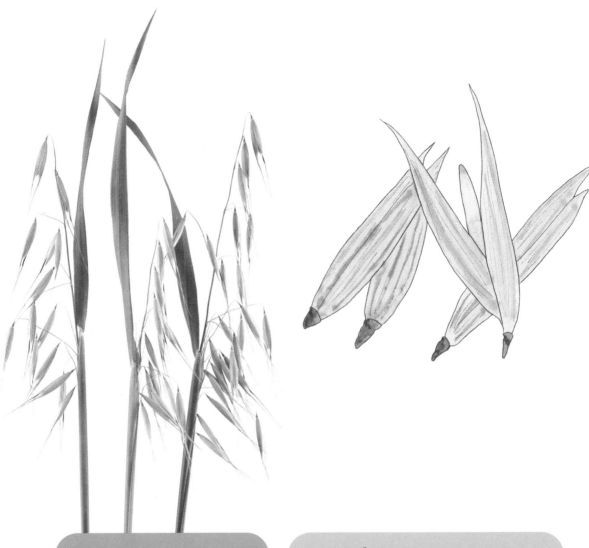

Musings

"Sowing our wild oats" is helpful for our libido and cardiac health. Associated with Earth goddesses for fertility and abundance, oatstraw activates our heart chakra. Known as one of the best remedies to provide nourishment for the nervous system, especially if we feel under stress.

Make

When your nerves feel frazzled, make a sweet milky tea with 1 to 2 tablespoons oatstraw to 1 cup (240 ml) water and milk combination. It combines well with lemon balm, stinging nettles, skullcap, chamomile, and passionflower. Create a bath ritual with a muslin bag full of oatstraw to relax your mind and promote tranquility. Use oatstraw in footbaths, facial scrubs, and dream pillows.

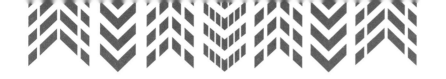

CHOKECHERRY

Prunus virginiana
Prunus virginiana var. *demissa*
Prunus virginiana var. *melanocarpa*
Prunus virginiana var. *virginiana*
Prunus virginiana var. *oregana*

My good sister and I have been asked to look over an Indigenous Welcome Garden at one of our local city pools. It was planted in 2013 with a diversity of native species, such as salmonberry, thimbleberry, hazelnut, red osier dogwood, snowberry, Oregon grape, strawberry, and a few chokecherry trees, all under the sentinel of a birch tree. Every visit we are greeted by the resident hummingbird, and in the late summer many birds are in the fruit trees, feasting. When the chokecherries are still hanging in the fall, the robins love to get a little tipsy from the intoxicating, fermented cherries.

In Daniel E. Moerman's book on ethnobotany, there are 1,649 species listed for food, with chokecherry being mentioned the most. I counted over fifty-seven different species under the *Prunus* genus entry in Daniel's book, an example of her deep relationship with our living world. The Navajo Ramah People considered chokecherry "life medicine," as she offers implements and the gift of stories to guide us to walk a good road. The Shoshone People made medicine spoons for their ceremonial Dog Feast. The Shuswap Nations mixed berries with bear grease for painting pictographs. The Dakota, Omaha, Pawnee, and Ponca saw the fruit as their seasonal indicator for the time of the Sun Dance.

Found in the understory, chokecherry grows from a large shrub into a small tree with broad, egg-shaped, pointed-edge leaves. Chokecherry's gray bark is covered with prominent lenticels, which are raised pores that allow gas exchange between internal tissues and our atmosphere. Scratch the branches to smell her "cherry cough syrup" aroma. The white flowers grow on racemes, ripening into berries for harvest in July or August.

All parts contain cyanide except the flesh of the cherry. The pea-size cherries have been described as ranging from tart and astringent to flavorful. I suspect the quality of the soil and the amount of sunlight contribute to the flavor. Chokecherry trees live from twenty to forty years and can yield up to 30 to 40 pounds (13.5 to 18 kg) per year of cherries, which are high in antioxidants and good fiber.

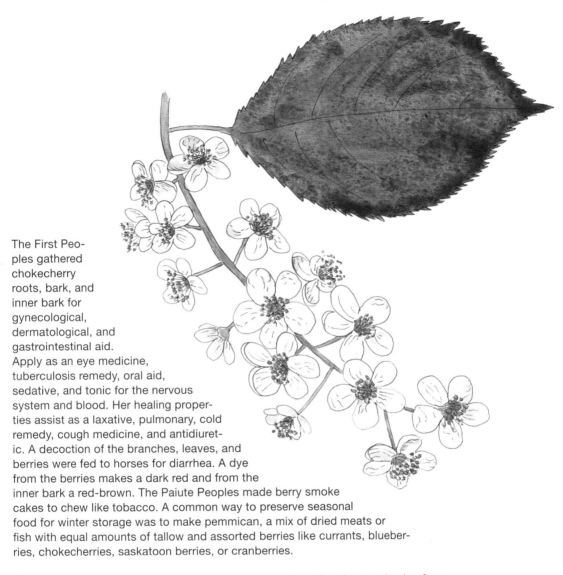

The First Peoples gathered chokecherry roots, bark, and inner bark for gynecological, dermatological, and gastrointestinal aid. Apply as an eye medicine, tuberculosis remedy, oral aid, sedative, and tonic for the nervous system and blood. Her healing properties assist as a laxative, pulmonary, cold remedy, cough medicine, and antidiuretic. A decoction of the branches, leaves, and berries were fed to horses for diarrhea. A dye from the berries makes a dark red and from the inner bark a red-brown. The Paiute Peoples made berry smoke cakes to chew like tobacco. A common way to preserve seasonal food for winter storage was to make pemmican, a mix of dried meats or fish with equal amounts of tallow and assorted berries like currants, blueberries, chokecherries, saskatoon berries, or cranberries.

Chokecherries are an important food for many animals such as bears, skunks, foxes, deer, moose, rabbits, and over seventy species of birds, such as robins, thrushes, jays, grosbeaks, woodpeckers, wild turkeys, scarlet tangiers, and grouse.

Pemmican is a unique preserved food that the Métis People made. Traditionally, buffalo meat was dried and pounded and mixed with an equal amount of tallow, a rendered animal fat, and an assortment of wild berries. Tallow greatly enhanced the pemmican's caloric and nutrient density.

continued on next page

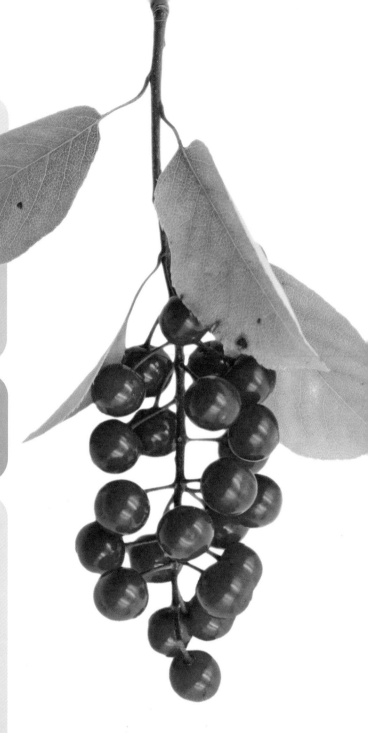

Look-alikes

Black cherry (*Prunus serotina*) has a rounded leaf edge.

Make

We can use the berries to make wine, beer, smoothies, syrup, jam, jellies, pies, and sauces.

Note

Chokecherry interacts with anticoagulants and antiplatelet drugs.

Musings

Sometimes we see contradictions in listings in which the same plant would be known to be a stimulant or a sedative. We may say an herb is poisonous or it might be used as an antidote for poisoning. In most societies, plant medicines were respected, potent, sometimes poisonous, and associated with strong powers in nature. In Daniel E. Moerman's book, *Native American Ethnobotany*, we are reminded that many medicines are toxic, best prescribed by a trained knowledge keeper. Remember, the poison is in the dose, so work with an experienced practitioner.

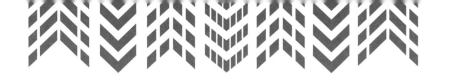

CALIFORNIA POPPY

Eschscholzia californica

It has been reported that in the1800s, various Tribes such as the Yakut and Pima applied California poppy for toothaches, teething, children's colic, and sleep. The roots act as a sedative and for the pain of shingles or sciatica. The flowers can be chewed as gum.

California poppy is easy to grow. She prefers a hot, dry space and can handle poor soil. The orange or yellow flowers grow in size based on how much water she receives. A wide range of bees love her pollen, although she lacks nectar. In a mild climate she may regrow for several years or reseed each year. Her bright orange flower closes on cloudy days and overnight. On occasion, I have found native bees resting in her closed flowers.

Both the flowers and the seeds can be eaten. Eat the flowers in salads or as garnishes and grind the seeds into powder for seasoning. She contains carotenoids, phytosterols, and alkaloids, promoting body and mind relaxation. California poppy attaches to the opioid receptors in our body and her hypnotic effects help us fall asleep faster or stay asleep, avoiding overnight awakenings. She is a great nervine and an antispasmodic.

Make

Make California poppy tea with the whole plant, fresh or dried. Collect when in full bloom, with flowers and the pink receptacle seedpods. It is always great to create a synergetic blend with lemon balm and passionflower. The whole plant can also be made into an alcohol tincture.

 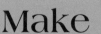

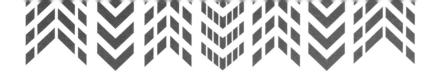

CATTAIL

Typha latifolia
Typha angustifolia
Typha domingensis
Typha x *glauca*

Common cattail is a gift that protects the shoreline from erosion, is a habitat for wildlife, provides shelter for birds and cover for fish, while attracting insects for fish to eat. Cattail traps sediment and silt, harboring microorganisms that break down organic waste like arsenic and removes polluting material. This landscape is a great reminder of how we make space for all of our relatives. When my daughter was young, I would take her to a local urban park to wave the wands of cattail spike heads, helping disperse the seeds.

There are many descriptions in *Native American Ethnobotany* of macerating and boiling the roots to make a fine syrup for sweet-ening or for cornmeal pudding, as the Haudenosaunee would make. Cattails' rhizomes were dried and ground into mush to make bread and flat cakes. Mature seed heads were burned to extract the seeds for gruel and soups. The pollen is used as a ceremonial face paint for many Tribes and Nations on Turtle Island. The list is endless for all the ways we can reengage with this relationship and rebuild our ponds and marshes that have been lost to development.

The Ojibwe People called cattail *apakwe* meaning, "put on a roof, final, cover a lodge." The leaves were important material for weaving baskets, hats, mats, and beds. The spikes would be dipped in animal fat to burn as a torch. Children's dolls were crafted and duck decoys were shaped from the leaves. Allowing for air movement, the seed fluff is an amazing insulation for boots, mittens, duvets, and the walls of the lodging.

In Euell Gibbons's book, *Stalking the Wild Asparagus*, he says to collect the young shoots, known as corms, when the stalks are around 2 feet (61 cm) high. Cattails are eaten raw or steamed with butter and are described as sweet and juicy with a cucumber-celery flavor. She contains potassium, phosphorus, and vitamins A, B, and C. The male is full of nutty-tasting, yellow pollen, which is easy to collect to make pancakes, cornbread, and muffins. It can also be added as an extender or thickener.

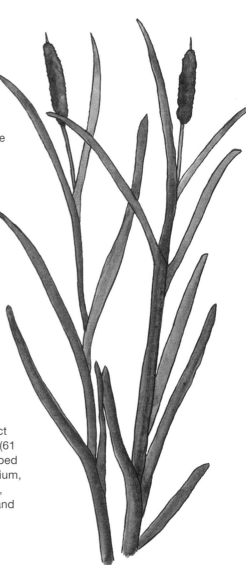

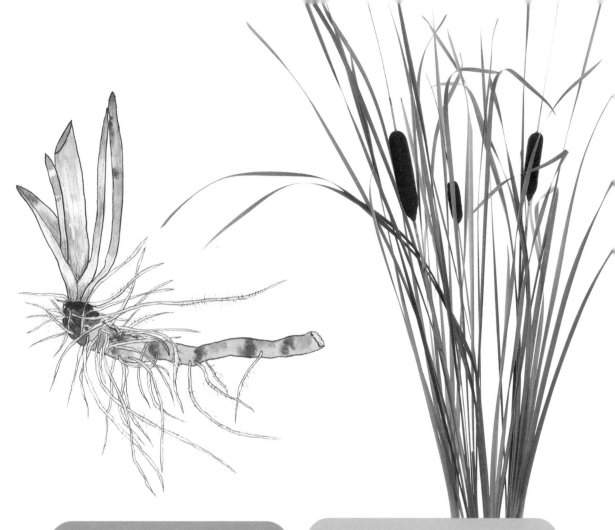

Make

Poultices can be made with the rhizomes for cuts, wounds, burns, insect stings, and bruises. The ash of the leaf is antiseptic and helps stop bleeding. Plus, a first aid gel is found between the leaf blades. This honey-like gel can be extracted and applied to wounds, scrapes, and toothaches. In Traditional Chinese Medicine, Pu Huang capsules are filled with pollen and used for nosebleeds, uterine bleeding, and blood in the urine.

Note

Do not use when pregnant.

Look-alikes

Poisonous blue flag iris (*Iris versicolor*) and yellow flag iris (*Iris pseudacorus*), the wild sedges in the Cyperaceae family, and sweet flag (*Acorus calamus*), which is an edible and medicinal, can be confused for cattail.

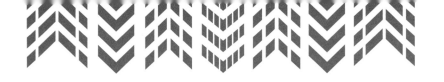

WILD BERGAMOT

Monarda didyma
Monarda fistulosa
Monarda fistulosa var. *menthifolia*

Monarda is grown as a honey source, an ornamental, and for her medicine. One of our native flowers here on Turtle Island, it has a long history with our Indigenous relatives from New York State who supplied "Liberty tea" during the Boston Tea Party conflict. Many of us may have been told that she is the one who flavors Earl Grey tea. The truth is that the flavor comes from the essential oils of Mediterranean citrus, *Citrus bergamia*.

The Cheyenne, Crow, Dakota, Kutenai, and Omaha created incense and fragrance with leaves placed on hot rocks in their sweat lodges and carried bunches of her aroma in their pockets. Wild bergamot was mixed with other aromatics, infused with beaver castor oil, and the perfume used on their hair, body, or clothing. She was collected for medicine to help with colds, flus, gingivitis, venomous bites, wounds, colic, gastrointestinal upset, and sweating. Her high thymol content makes her a good choice for a respiratory tea or a strong infusion used as mouthwash.

Monarda has a diversity of flavors, with a range of subtleties and heat. Her scent has been described as lemony and sweet to hot and spicy. When you rub the leaves, you will smell the fragrance of oregano. Our Indigenous Relatives flavored their meat with monarda and used her as a food preservative. The flavor of *Monarda fistulosa* var. *menthifolia* is great for spaghetti, venison stew, salsa, hot sauce, burritos, beans, and pizza.

Both the flower and the leaves are edible. Collect the leaves before the flower blooms. Cut the flowers just above the nodes and hang them to dry in bundles of four or five stalks out of the sunlight for a few weeks. When properly dried and stored, monarda retains a high concentration of volatile oils. Most delicate herbs can be stored for one year, but monarda can be stored for up to two years.

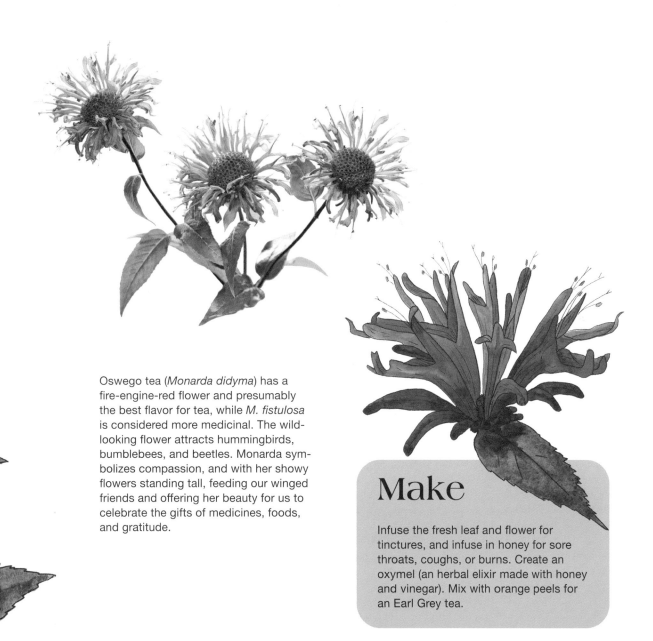

Oswego tea (*Monarda didyma*) has a fire-engine-red flower and presumably the best flavor for tea, while *M. fistulosa* is considered more medicinal. The wild-looking flower attracts hummingbirds, bumblebees, and beetles. Monarda symbolizes compassion, and with her showy flowers standing tall, feeding our winged friends and offering her beauty for us to celebrate the gifts of medicines, foods, and gratitude.

Make

Infuse the fresh leaf and flower for tinctures, and infuse in honey for sore throats, coughs, or burns. Create an oxymel (an herbal elixir made with honey and vinegar). Mix with orange peels for an Earl Grey tea.

Steaming bergamot is a powerful way to clear congestion. Boil water in a soup pot, one-third full, then add four or five flower heads and a handful of leaf. Infuse for 10 minutes. Place the soup pot with the lid on the floor and sit with your head above the pot. Cover yourself with a bed sheet and slowly open the pot lid a small crack to allow the steam to rise so you do not feel overwhelmed by the heat and aroma. Close your eyes and slowly breathe through your mouth. Play soothing music and ask for healing in your prayers. Should the steam be too spicy, cover the soup pot and take a break. It is suggested to steam three times over the course of the day. You can also do a footbath.

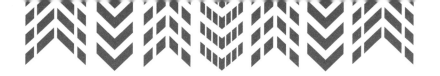

CATNIP

Nepeta cataria

Catnip is a member of the mint family, which explains why she is fast-growing. However, she is more drought tolerant than some of her thirsty mint cousins. She has heart-shaped, oval-toothed, gray-green leaves and a square stem covered with fine hairs. The *Nepeta* genus produces a compound called nepetalactone, a chemical similar to a feline pheromone that activates the momentary craziness we witness when cats smell her. You might find her scent a little pungent and skunky, which is a reason why she is planted as a companion herb to keep rodents and rabbits out of the garden. Collect the leaf and flower to use fresh or dried.

Catnip helps with digestion, soothes intestinal cramps, increases appetite, induces menstruation, helps migraines, eases anxiety, and relieves colds and fevers. She is a strong gastrointestinal antispasmodic and considered one of the best remedies for stress-induced irritable bowel syndrome. Consume catnip in small amounts.

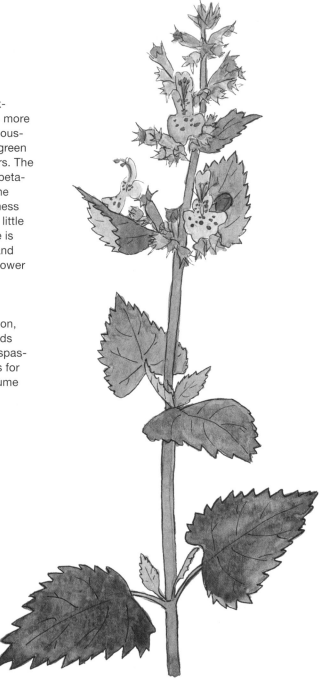

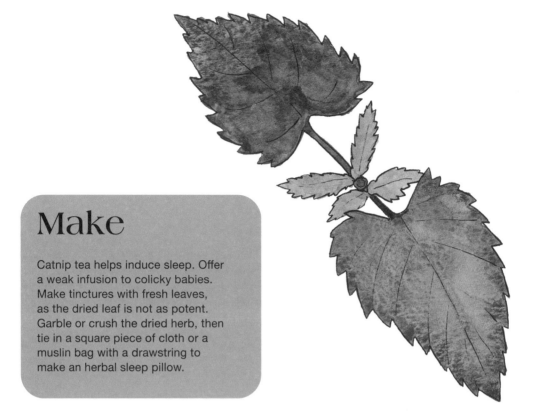

Make

Catnip tea helps induce sleep. Offer a weak infusion to colicky babies. Make tinctures with fresh leaves, as the dried leaf is not as potent. Garble or crush the dried herb, then tie in a square piece of cloth or a muslin bag with a drawstring to make an herbal sleep pillow.

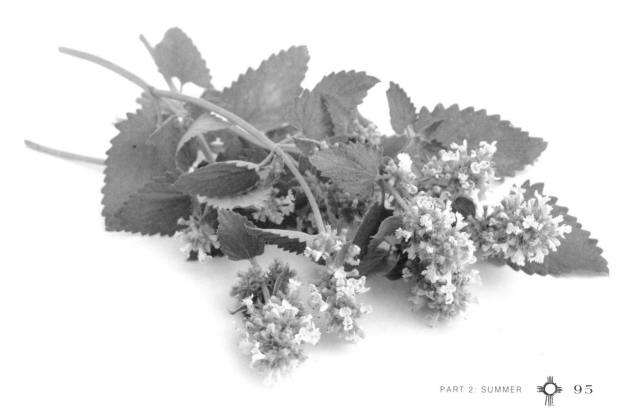

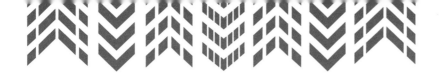

PEPPERMINT

Mentha piperita
Mentha longifolia

Mary Siisip Geniusz was the Woman of the Northwest Wind, an Anishinaabe/ Ojibwe medicine woman, ethnobotanist, professor at the University of Wisconsin- Milwaukee, and apprentice of Keewaydinoquay. Her book, *Plants Have So Much to Give Us, All We Have to Do Is Ask*, is a rich account of our relationships with our More-Than-Human-Kin who carry their own stories, teachings, and way of life. In the Anishinaabe protocols, they are required to introduce plants as we would another human being. As we get to know plants, we develop a fondness for a specific plant. For Keewaydinoquay, it was mint, which she added to everything. Mint can be added to cookies, smoking mix, anointing oils, skin creams, bathwater, candles, soups, and (something I never considered) coffee.

Mints are best grown in containers as they like to travel in the garden! While some may call her invasive, my sense is that she is looking for more nutrients. Feed her rich compost and hopefully she will stay put and be grateful for the food.

Engage with all of your senses when identifying mint; smell and taste a little. She has the distinguished square stem, with her flowers growing in whorls around the stem. Little joints at the nodes can easily grow when placed in water, making her easy to propagate. Mint loves water, so make sure she has enough moisture.

Peppermint offers many varieties like spearmint, orange mint, apple mint, pineapple mint, and chocolate mint, a favorite tea. None in the mint family are poisonous except pennyroyal (*Hedeoma pulegioides*), identifiable because she does not emit the aroma of other mints with her leaf.

Cultivated in Europe and America for her aerial parts, *Mentha piperita* is used in the essential oil industry. Essential oils are very potent medicines and should be used with great care. When chemical compounds are isolated they have the potential to harm, hence why we want the whole plant to balance out the pure oil's potency. She contains menthol, menthyl acetate, piperitone, limonene, cineole, pulegone, and a- and b-pinene. Insect repellents can be manufactured with isolated pulegone, the active chemical compound found in pennyroyal. Studies have shown a link to liver cancers when pulegone is absorbed through the skin.

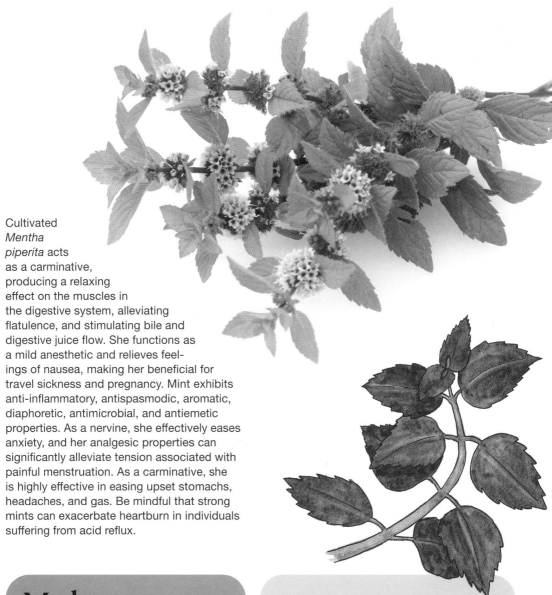

Cultivated *Mentha piperita* acts as a carminative, producing a relaxing effect on the muscles in the digestive system, alleviating flatulence, and stimulating bile and digestive juice flow. She functions as a mild anesthetic and relieves feelings of nausea, making her beneficial for travel sickness and pregnancy. Mint exhibits anti-inflammatory, antispasmodic, aromatic, diaphoretic, antimicrobial, and antiemetic properties. As a nervine, she effectively eases anxiety, and her analgesic properties can significantly alleviate tension associated with painful menstruation. As a carminative, she is highly effective in easing upset stomachs, headaches, and gas. Be mindful that strong mints can exacerbate heartburn in individuals suffering from acid reflux.

Make

Mint is best served cold for the most effective medicine. Infuse her leaves in hot water for 10 to 15 minutes, then let the tea cool before drinking. As a tonic and stimulant, add mint to salads, stir-fries, jams, jellies, sauces, stuffing, ice cream, and lemonade. Chop fresh mint, add to water, and freeze in ice cube trays.

Stephanie Rose's book *Garden Alchemy* uses plant medicine as garden medicine. Her recipe for a natural insect repellent is useful to deter ants, aphids, cabbage loopers, flea beetles, squash bugs, and whiteflies. Blend 6 garlic cloves, 1 or 2 whole chile peppers with seeds, ½ cup (15 g) chopped mint leaves, 1 cup (240 ml) water, and ¼ teaspoon liquid castile soap. Strain through a nut milk bag and add to a spray bottle to repel insects.

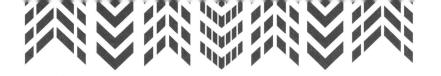

GARDEN SAGE

Salvia officinalis

Our wild sages, *Salvia apiana*, are now classified as an endangered species, according to the Airmid Institue, which reports on at-risk flora and advocates "protecting medicinal and aromatic plants—and their use in traditional medicine—for future generations." Our Indigenous brothers and sisters work to regenerate, protect, and preserve our wild sage. All of us can help by considering garden sage (*S. officinalis*) for smudging. *Salvia* is a Latin verb meaning "to save," and *officinalis* notes that is it an official medicinal herb. Garden sage is filled with the herbal, spicy, and earthy aromas of resin and eucalyptus.

Garden sage is a common member in our Mediterranean herb garden. She tolerates dry, free-draining soil, loves the sun, prefers a sheltered spot, and can be grown in containers. She is a perennial evergreen, with grayish leaves, a woody stem, and stunning blue to purplish flowers. A cousin of mint, both in the Lamiaceae family, she contains chlorogenic, caffeic, rosmarinic, and ellagic acids that work as antioxidants. These chemical constituents help lower cancer risk as well as aiding in brain function and memory. She is a source of bioactive calcium, relieving the pain of joint aches. Garden sage is said to transform grief and depression and help us age with grace, hardiness, and humor.

Smudging is an ancient Indigenous sacred ceremonial practice for purification. Cleansing is another practice in which many cultures around the world burn herbs to cleanse their homes and environments. Research has shown that cleansing hinders bacteria in the air, repels insects, helps improve mood, and reduces stress. Collect garden sage, lavender, rosemary, along with other aromatics, bundle the fresh herbs together, tie with hemp thread, and hang to dry. You only need a few leaves to cleanse.

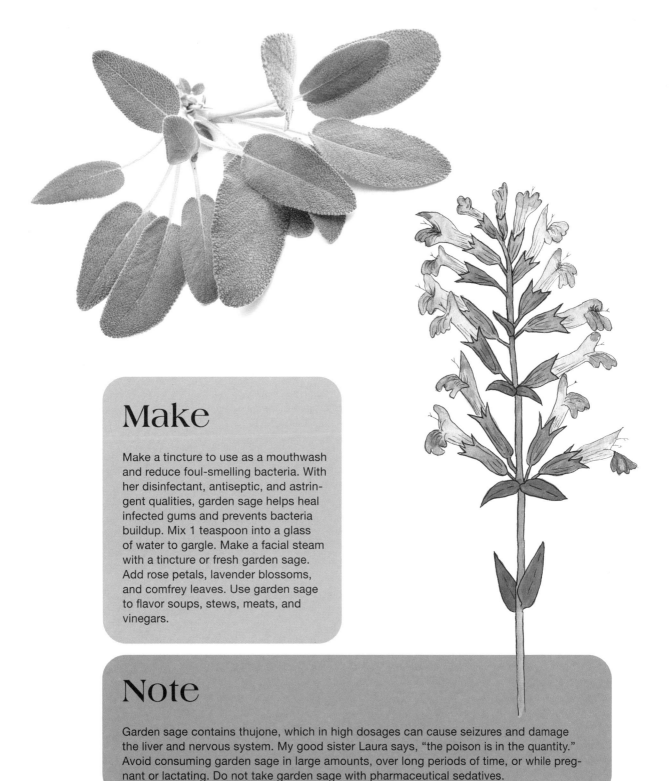

Make

Make a tincture to use as a mouthwash and reduce foul-smelling bacteria. With her disinfectant, antiseptic, and astringent qualities, garden sage helps heal infected gums and prevents bacteria buildup. Mix 1 teaspoon into a glass of water to gargle. Make a facial steam with a tincture or fresh garden sage. Add rose petals, lavender blossoms, and comfrey leaves. Use garden sage to flavor soups, stews, meats, and vinegars.

Note

Garden sage contains thujone, which in high dosages can cause seizures and damage the liver and nervous system. My good sister Laura says, "the poison is in the quantity." Avoid consuming garden sage in large amounts, over long periods of time, or while pregnant or lactating. Do not take garden sage with pharmaceutical sedatives.

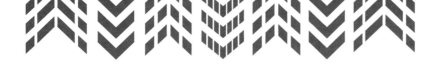

ROSEMARY

Salvia rosmarinus

Rosemary was first mentioned as a medicine on cuneiform stone tablets dating back to 5000 BCE. She arrived on Turtle Island in the seventeenth century and is now found globally. The ancient Greeks dedicated rosemary to Aphrodite. Rosemary crowns were adorned on the heads of brides for love and fertility. As a folklore medicine, rosemary is known to alleviate headaches, stomachaches, epilepsy, rheumatic pain, depression, and nervous disorders and improve memory. She is anti-inflammatory, antioxidant, neuroprotective, and antidepressive. Today, we understand the role of free radicals and oxidative stress in the aging process, and these markers are connected to cognitive decline and Alzheimer's disease. Her aerosols of essential oils have an effect on our moods, help with studying and recall, and decrease cortisol levels. Rosemary is a great natural sleep aid for dreaming, supporting memory, and recalling dreams.

One of her many benefits is to help with hair loss. Compared with its essential oil, the plant itself contains a wide spectrum of lipid-soluble antioxidants, polyphenols, and fatty acids. Olive oil infused with rosemary will stimulate the hair follicles, improving hair growth and increasing circulation to the scalp. Compared to commercial medications, rosemary-infused oil can be more effective at reducing hair loss.

Here on the West Coast, our winters are very mild, and we can witness our perennial evergreen, drought-resistant rosemary in bloom before any other flowers in the early spring. It is a gift to see her beautiful purplish blue flowers showing on cool gray days. Her former (now synonym) Latin name, *Rosmarinus*, refers to the "dew of the sea."

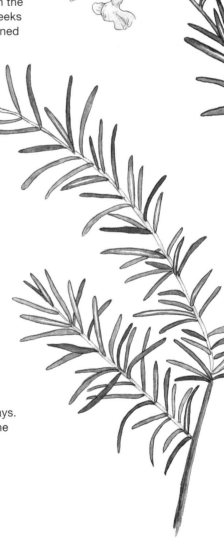

Make

Steep tea for a hair rinse and pour into spray bottles to apply. A hair rinse is not recommended for those who suffer from hormonal effects, older folks, or those with dandruff that might be caused by inflammation and irritation. Make a hair oil with 75 percent rosemary-infused olive oil and 25 percent castor oil, as castor oil is rich in oleic acid and omega-6 fatty acids, supporting stronger, thicker hair. Apply twice a week and leave on overnight, covering the head with a shower cap. If it is too stimulating, leave on for an hour and wash out. Use sparingly. Add rosemary leaf to a dream pillow or put a sprig under your pillow to ward off nightmares.

Musings

Herbs that are mostly water-soluble have fewer side effects and fewer complications than herbs that are not water-soluble. That said, they can still be powerful medicine. I once made a tea with two leaves of rosemary and was surprised how stimulating she is for circulation! It was strong for me, but maybe not for you. Research and experiment. Listen to your body to discover how an herb can be your medicine.

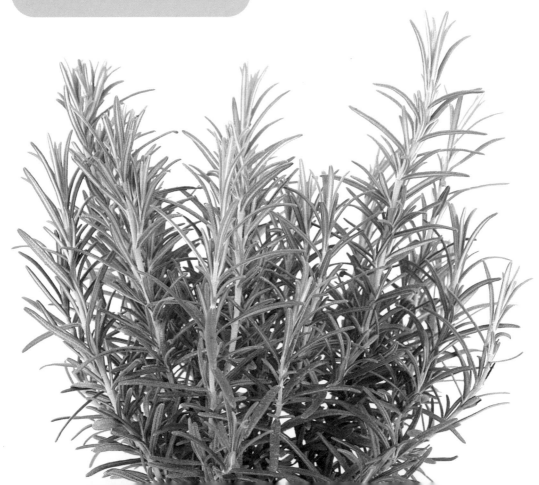

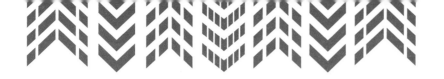

LEMON BALM

Melissa officinalis

My herb teacher Don would say, "Whoever is growing around you is your medicine." My former partner would say, "You make a great doctor but a terrible patient." Where we lived raising our daughters in the city, we had abundant lemon balm growing around the house. Known as a nervine, lemon balm is helpful for my nervous system.

Cultivated and used in Iran, lemon balm is a medicine for digestion, pain, and nerves. Traditional uses include tranquilizing, fever-reducing, memory-enhancing, menstruation-inducing, thyroid treatment. She is widely known to be helpful for headaches and insomnia. Lemon balm extracts have been reported to reduce systolic and diastolic blood pressure. She may affect thyroid function as she reduces hormone levels and will interfere with thyroid hormone replacement. She is one of the easiest herbs to grow, especially for a beginner gardener, but keep in mind she spreads readily.

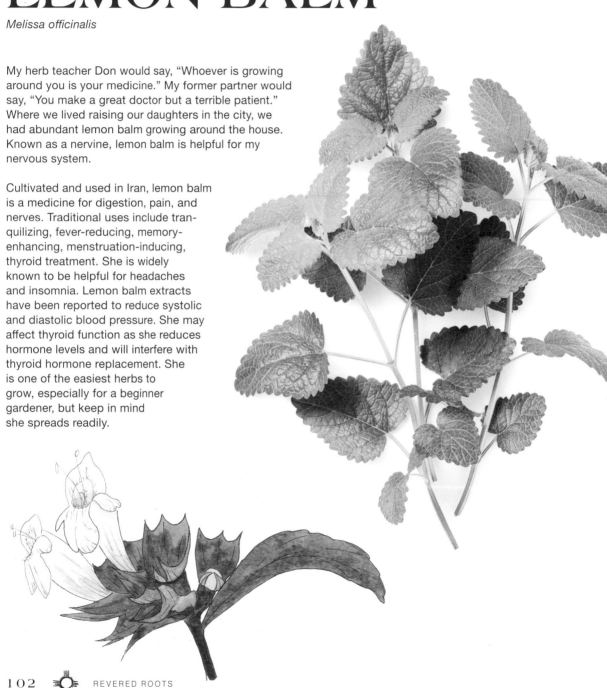

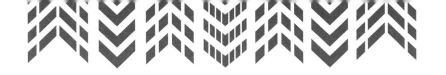

WILLOW

Salix species

I rarely find willow here in our city. Down by the river on the lands of the Musqueam People, there is a Grandmother Willow who stretches out across a little creek, protecting the water from Grandfather Sun. In the early spring, as the catkins open and expand, a diversity of life is buzzing around her. Willow loves wet areas and cool climates, and her bark, twigs, and leaf have gifted us with natural healing since ancient times. Clay tablets from the Assyrians in the Sumerian period around four thousand years ago prescribed willow leaves for rheumatic disease. Egyptians used her for joint pain and inflammation, and Hippocrates recommended willow bark extraction for fever, pain, and childbirth. Willow is Nature's pain reliever.

We find evidence from the ancient Chinese, Romans, and our Native American civilizations recognizing the benefits of willow, which contains salicylates, medicine for pain relief. Salicylates in herbs include compounds of salicin, methyl salicylate, and salicylic acid. These phytohormones activate plant growth and seed germination, root initiation, stomatal closure, transpiration, floral activation, photosynthesis, and plant immunity. These phytohormones also signal defense against pathogens along with other processes. The volatile ester of methyl salicylate signals other More-Than-Human-Kin within the forest for mutual immunity.

Salicin, the active ingredient found in willow, is converted into salicylic acid, which interacts with enzymes and bacterial gut flora when indigested via teas or tinctures. The body uses it as an analgesic, anti-inflammatory, antiseptic, and antirheumatic agent. It has slower absorption than a synthetic, promotes more dispersal within the body, lasts longer, and is better tolerated because it does not upset the stomach lining. That said, it is not pleasant tasting.

continued on next page

Salicin is also an ingredient in many skin care products as the keratolytic and comedolytic compounds cause the cells of the skin to shed more readily, opening closed pores, neutralizing bacteria, and making room for more cell growth. High dosages of salicylic acid has been known to create hearing loss in zinc-deficient individuals as it inhibits the motor protein prestin in the cochlea area of the ear. Overdose of salicylates can produce toxicity symptoms of abdominal pain, nausea, vomiting, dizziness, tinnitus, and tiredness.

Salicylic acid is made up of two groups, the phenol (OH) group and the carboxylic acid (COOH) group. Many doctors worked to synthesize carboxylic acid, which they discovered irritates the stomach and has an unpleasant taste. Around 1897, Dr. Hoffmann managed to synthesize it from the phenol group, and for the first time successfully created a synthetic drug: aspirin. *A* for "acetyl" and *spir* from the herb *Filipendula* (syn. *Spiraea*) *ulmaria*, known as meadowsweet. This spearheaded the industry of animal testing and the pharmaceutical trade. Salicin does not affect the antiplatelet reaction like aspirin does.

Harvest willow bark and twigs after the leaves have fallen and before the buds swell in early spring. The ideal conditions are when the ground is frozen. Use fresh when making herbal alcohol tinctures. For an herbal tea, infuse fresh or dried willow.

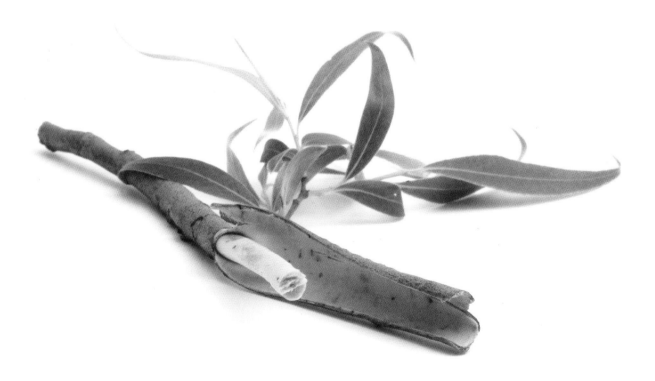

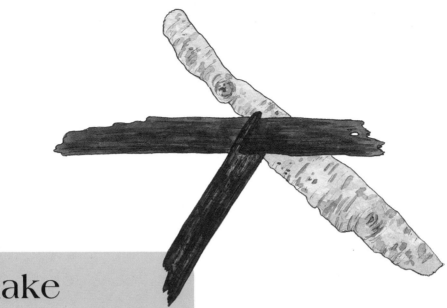

Make

The book *Medical Herbalism* by David Hoffmann suggests making a decoction with willow using 1 to 2 teaspoons in 1 cup (240 ml) water. Bring to a boil and simmer for 10 to 15 minutes and steep another 30 minutes. Drink three times daily. For an alcohol tincture, infuse a ratio of one part either fresh or dried willow bark to five parts 25 to 40 percent alcohol and steep 4 to 6 weeks. Strain, bottle, and label. Take ½ to 1 teaspoon three times daily.

Musings

Willow is associated with the Greek goddess Hecate, who is linked to the moon and water. Willow symbolizes our capacity to withstand hardship, survive loss, and rebirth through difficult emotions.

Medicines to Help Us, a collection of the teachings of Métis Elder Rose Richardson, and featuring Christi Belcourt's artwork, reminds us of our responsibility. We have a lifetime of learning protocols and deep commitment to Creator. Healing is represented in the four directions of the Medicine Wheel: our mental, emotional, spiritual, and physical bodies. Herbs can be gentle and toxic. One medicine does not fit all bodies.

Forty species of willow are mentioned in Daniel E. Moerman's book, *Native American Ethnobotany*, ranging from medicinal uses to ceremonial applications. In traditional Indigenous ways, healing is holistically approached. It is understood that our existence is deeply tied to our kinship between our relatives of the Rooted Nations. We live in a continual reality, through ceremonies activating the interconnectiveness with our bodies, the plant medicines, and the Spirit world. This is a personal experience, as our spiritual practices are not shared publicly.

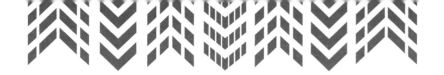

ALFALFA

Medicago sativa

In Arabic cultures, alfalfa was considered the "father of all foods." The Chinese ingested her as an appetite stimulant and our Indigenous relatives applied her to stimulate blood clotting, gain energy, and strengthen bones. She is a superfood, an easy-to-grow perennial from the legume family. Grown for livestock and cover crops, alfalfa has a taproot that can grow 60 feet (18 m) down into Mother Earth, making her drought tolerant. Her life span is four to five years. Collect the top one-third of the plant when she is 2 to 6 feet (61 cm to 1.8 m) tall and in full bloom. Her seeds can be sprouted as a super nutritious green. Alfalfa is high in nutrients, minerals, trace minerals, enzymes, proteins, carotenoids, calcium, chlorophyll, and vitamins A, B, C, D, E, and K. She improves the appetite and lowers cholesterol and plaque in the arteries.

Alfalfa's leaf is antibacterial, diuretic, and laxative and helps our bodies recuperate after an illness. She is anti-inflammatory and lowers pain, especially for PMS and headaches. Alfalfa benefits healthy skin, reduces ulcers, and nourishes bone and joint disorders. She tones the kidneys, is a blood cleanser, treats urinary tract infections, and helps with menopause symptoms. Alfalfa is known to bring endometriosis relief, increase breast milk, and decrease allergies. She is detoxifying and antiseptic, improves liver function, and provides iron without inducing constipation.

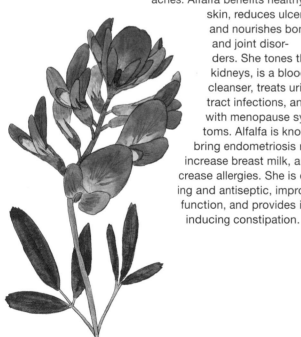

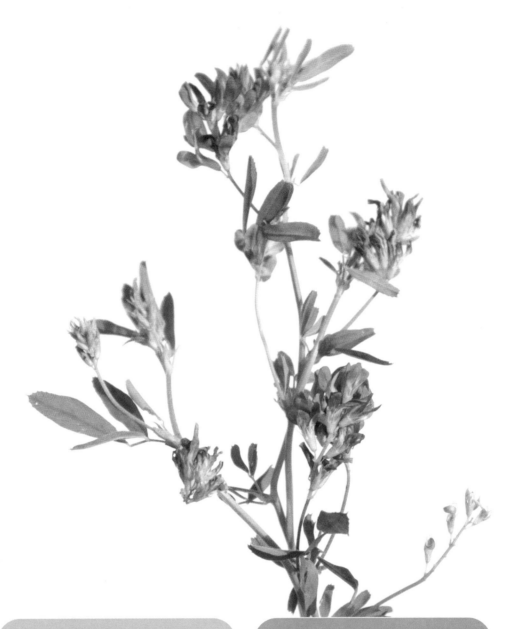

Make

Place 2 tablespoons (16 g) alfalfa seeds in a clean jar with a cheese-cloth cover held in place with a rubber band. Rinse and drain the seeds in the jar two times a day until sprouted, usually within 3 to 4 days.

Note

Don't take alfalfa with vitamin E as her saponins interfere with absorption. Also, avoid alfalfa if you have auto-immune diseases like lupus. She also contains vitamin K, which interferes with anticoagulants.

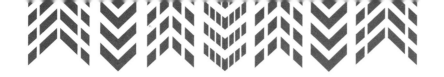

CALENDULA

Calendula officinalis

Worldwide, we find many garden benefits when calendula is grown in community with other More-Than-Human-Kin. She can be grown as a cover crop for early spring blooming flowers. Her roots aid the soil by forming a symbiotic relationship with soil fungi. She is very helpful for soil restoration requiring cadmium. Described as living mulch, calendula enriches the soil with her biomass. Through observation, we see that she enhances fruit tree guilds to attract pollinators and as a "trap crop" for aphids, whiteflies, mites, and thrips, which become trapped in her sticky resin.

Calendula extracts have reduced tobacco cutworms. Grown alongside cabbage, she deters aphids and diamondback moths. She is also known to repel worms in tomatoes and various nematodes. Her nectar feeds butterflies, goldenrod spiders, lacewings, sweat bees, bumblebees, hoverflies, and honeybees. One cool fall morning I was collecting her flower heads from my patio pots and I discovered a little native bee curled up in her closed flower. Calendula also hosts an attractive space for ladybugs.

A common name for calendula is pot marigold, although marigolds fall under the genus of *Tagetes*, an herbaceous plant native to southern Mexico. The spatulate or oblanceolate leaves are waxy, sticky, and aromatic, not found in the cultivars. Bright orange or yellow daisy-like monoecious flowers (either female or male and sometimes with both sexes on the same plant) grow up to 3 inches (7.5 cm) across. Both the ray florets and disk flower heads are held by a green bract. The ray petals have a little notch at the tip. Blooming from spring to the first heavy frost, calendula is a great cut flower and blooms more often when snipped. The flowers of calendula are edible and chickens love to eat them. You will notice that the eggs of hens fed calendula have a bright orange yolk, indicating high beta-carotene content.

Calendula is known for her healing abilities. She is antiseptic, antibacterial, anti-inflammatory, antiviral, and antimicrobial. She is mucilage, containing saponins, organic acids, enzymes, and resins. Calendula can improve circulation for skin ulcers, burns, and bruising and reduces scarring. She helps with itchy skin, diaper rash, bug bites, pink eye, varicose veins, sunburn, sinus infections, dandruff, and postpartum symptoms. She supports our liver, is diaphoretic to help reduce the temperature of fevers, activates a stagnant lymphatic system, and helps fight the infection of mastitis. Note that some folks may have allergies to calendula.

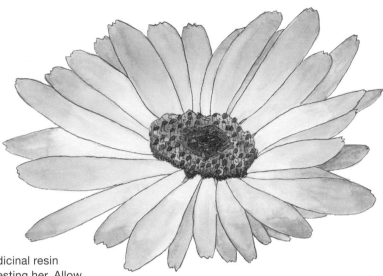

Collect calendula flowers in the morning after the dew is gone and the flowers have just opened. You will feel her sticky medicinal resin on your fingers when harvesting her. Allow the flowers to wilt overnight, then infuse the whole flower head, including the green bracts. Dried calendula flowers will only last up to 6 months. Store the dried plants in paper bags to avoid moisture contamination. If you live in a humid environment, it might be best to use a dehydrator. The shape of her seeds reminds me of little dinosaurs. Collect them to share with your neighbors or be a guerrilla gardener and toss the seeds in wild or abandoned spaces to add life and to support our pollinators.

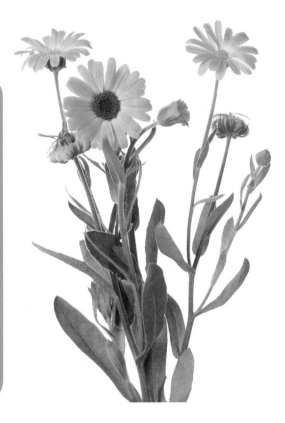

Make

Steep calendula flowers in tea to use as a gargle for sore throats. Make a strong antiseptic for wounds by pressing the flowers into fresh juice and applying it directly to scrapes, corns, or warts. Make a strong decoction using 1 ounce (28 g) herb in 1 quart (940 ml) boiling water and infuse for 4 to 8 hours. Consume the decoction slowly throughout the day, as she is bitter and may upset your stomach. Try an overnight decoction and warm it up in the morning with a little maple syrup to counteract the bitterness. Make a syrup with elderberry, ginger, orange peel, and calendula flower petals. When infusing into oils, she can be a bit tricky so make sure you dry the petals for a few days beforehand.

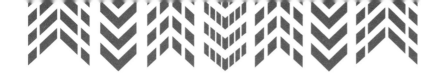

CORN SILK

Zea mays

Gardening invites us to be part of the great circle of life. Our relative, corn, symbolizes fertility and, for a long time in some parts of the world is acknowledged with great celebrations. She was adapted from a wild grass, *Teosinte*, "mother of the corn," from the Aztec language Nahuatl. The Mayan People were the first to breed the grass and by the 1600s the European settlers were shown how to plant the three sisters of corn, squash, and beans. The three sisters is a community guild of relatives better equipped to adapt with the ever-changing world when planted together, fostering collaboration and cooperation.

I was surprised to learn two decades ago that corn silk could be made into a tea and helps heal bladder infections. Corn silk relieves water retention from kidney disease, PMS, cystitis, and urinary and prostate infections. She soothes bladder irritation and reduces frequent urination. Corn is sweet, astringent, cooling, drying, moistening, nourishing, restoring, stimulating, dissolving, and softening. She is helpful with acute and chronic inflammation of the bladder.

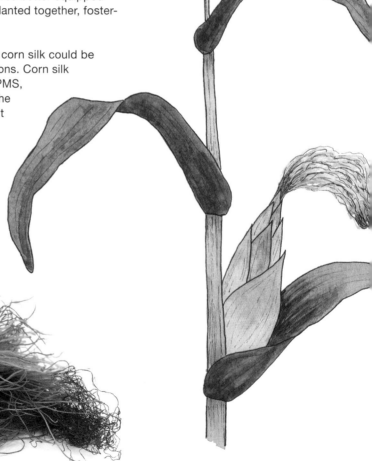

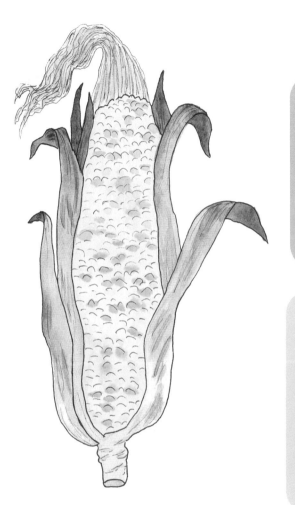

Make

Steep tea using 1 to 2 teaspoons in 1 to 2 quarts (1 to 1.8 L) water and drink 1 cup (240 ml) every hour for acute conditions. Make an alcohol tincture of one part plant to five parts 25 percent alcohol and take ½ teaspoon to 1 tablespoon (3 to 15 ml) per day.

An Indian scholar and founder of Navdanya, a movement for biodiversity conservation and farmers' rights, Vandana Shiva speaks on behalf of seeds. Seeds create renewal to be shared and dispersed. Seeds are our ancestors; they hold an ancient genetic code and are life itself. Let's be seed keepers again and share kindness and generosity in the public commons. Saving seeds is a promise to our ancestors to share a sacred covenant. Saving seeds of diversity is vital.

Rowen White, an Indigenous Mohawk/Kanienkeha:ka seed steward who weaves stories of ancestral foods and culture, says that seeds are a living, loving prayer in action. We sing the seeds awake when planting with the growing waxing moon. The gravitational pull brings the deep waters in Mother Earth to the surface to help germinate the seeds. The circle of life is the act of giving and receiving. Without us, there is no corn.

Musings

Basking in the sun with a dear sister while meditating on the shimmering sunlight on the Salish Sea, it came to me that we are made of sunlight. When we eat real food from the earth, we are eating light. Let food be your medicine and let medicine be your food.

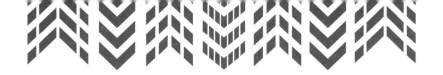

PASSIONFLOWER

Passiflora incarnata

Grown by the Aztec and Inca Peoples, passionflower was introduced to Europe in the late 1600s. One of the most fascinating and complexly evolved flowers, passionflower is native to the southeast region of Turtle Island. A perennial climbing vine, she prefers shade or partial shade with no full sun, slightly acidic soil that is rich and loamy, and plenty of water. All aerial parts and fruit are collected during the growing season.

The symbolic relationship with other Relatives like ants and butterflies is another example of the reciprocal interconnection that is paramount for evolution. Passionflower produces extrafloral nectaries, nectar-producing glands located throughout her leaves, flower buds, and stems. She attracts ants, who in return protect her from being eaten by other Creepy Crawlers. Passionflower is the only food sources for the Gulf fritillary (*Agraulis vanillae*) and variegated fritillary (*Euptoieta claudia*) caterpillars. Ants play a role to keep the garden in balance and have been witnessed collecting caterpillar eggs, and then replacing them on the passionflower.

Sometimes known as maypop, her name derived from *mahcawq* of the Powhatan People or *machkak* of the Menominee People. Traditionally, the Cherokee made medicine from the roots for boils and earaches and a beverage from the fruits. The Houma infused the roots as a tonic to cleanse the blood. Today, herbalists use only the leaves, stems, and flowers. Collect these parts when the leaves are green and vital. Her yellow, wrinkly fruit is edible, offering a sweet-sour flavor.

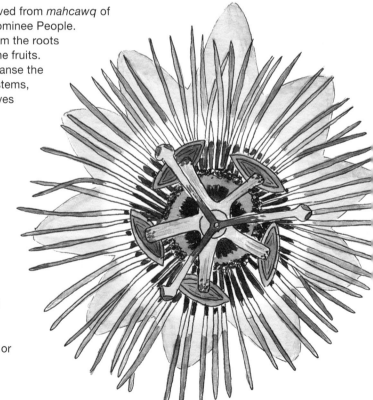

Containing alkaloids, passionflower can interfere with the production of monoamine oxidase, enzymes that remove neurotransmitters like norepinephrine, dopamine, and serotonin, as antidepressants do. She also contains gamma-aminobutyric acid (GABA). Found in the brain, GABA properties reduce blood pressure, decrease the effects of menopause, treat insomnia, reduce anger, and ease headaches. She offers many benefits in supporting withdrawal from opiates and benzodiazepines, and is helpful for epilepsy and ADHD. Passionflower has been used to reduce anxiety for patients going into surgery or undergoing dental extractions.

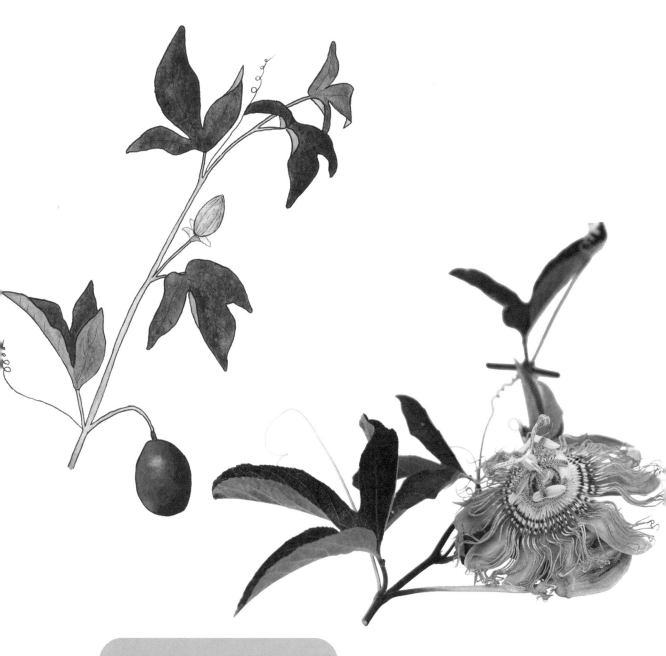

Make

Steep a tea of her dried leaf and combine with St. John's wort and valerian (*Valeriana officinalis*). Passionflower will potentiate medications and enhances the potency of St. John's wort.

Note

Not all species of passionflower are used for medicine. Reach out to a local herbalist, do your research, and grow your own.

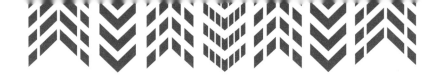

ELDERBERRY

Sambucus racemosa
Sambucus pubens var. *arborescens*
Sambucus cerulea

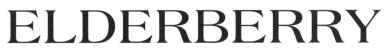

I remember a good friend sharing his excitement as the red elderberry flowers bloomed in the spring. He expressed his longing and memories of the time when his village would go out collecting. I long for a time when we have more of our native More-Than-Human-Kin surrounding us. Folks like to gather her delicate cluster of creamy white flowers to make into spring cordials. The small, seedy, red berry is an important food for the Central and Northern Nations of the coastal peoples. Archaeological sites found stored caches of berries dating back hundreds of years. Elderberries are considered a sacred herb to plant in your yard for good luck.

Sambucus cerulea, or blue elderberries, can be eaten fresh or cooked. You might notice a white bloom covering the berry, which is an epicuticular wax that protects the berries from UV rays and moisture loss. Flower clusters can be dipped in batter and fried, but only eat small amounts. In Europe, tea is made from the flowers for colds, flus, and fevers. She is known to stimulate urination and bowel movements, and the dried flowers can be used to wash hemorrhoids. Elderberry is diaphoretic and antiviral. Her berries are rich in many vitamins and minerals and can produce a crimson or violet dye. You can also crush her leaf and rub it on your skin as an insect repellent. All parts of the plant are toxic except for the flowers and the flesh of the berry. The safest way to prepare the berries is to cook the fruit.

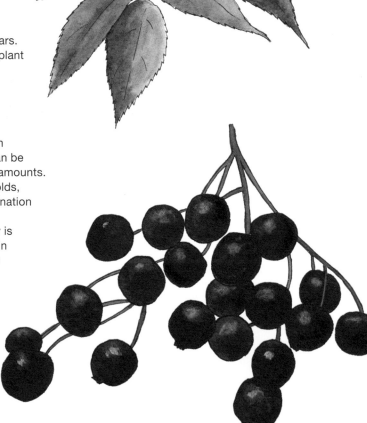

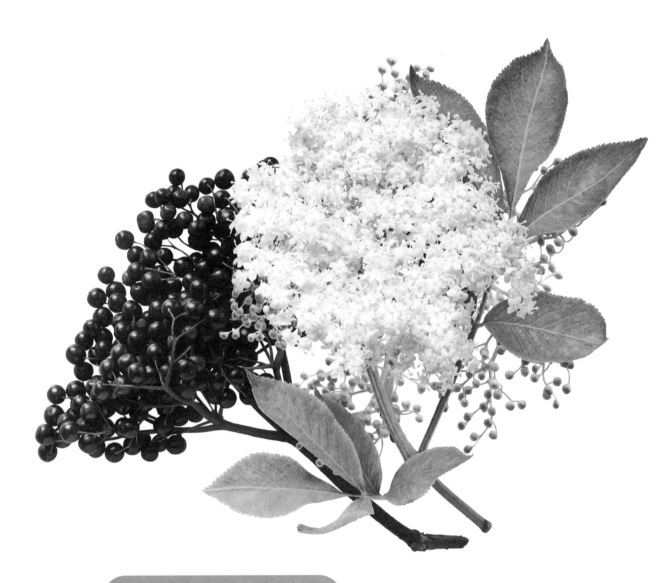

Make

Steep the berries for a refreshing tea, combining mint and yarrow. The berries and flowers make a tangy jam, sweet syrup, liqueurs, or wine.

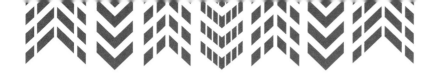

FEVERFEW

Tanacetum parthenium

A native from across the Atlantic Ocean, feverfew is found widely spread on Turtle Island and Australia. A short-lived perennial blooming from July to October, she emits a strong, bitter odor. Yellow-green leaves are alternate, growing on both sides of the stem. Bright, small, daisy-like flowers are arranged in dense flat-top clusters.

I love to sit, listen, and learn with other teachers about their experiences with herbs. Paul Bergner founded and teaches at the North American Institute of Medical Herbalism. Paul teaches about the six dimensions of medical herbs based on observations of how the herbs interact with us. The long history of Traditional Chinese Medicine (TCM) and Indian Ayurveda medicine also base their practices on energetics of herbs and people. How do they taste? What is their temperature? Humidity? What is the tone of the herb? Do they relax the tissue or firm it up? What tissue or body system do they have an affinity to? What are their clinical actions? Paul has been compiling data from his students based on their observations for over twenty years. It was interesting to hear Paul say how many women noted that feverfew disrupted their menstrual cycle. Feverfew is warm and dry in her energetics, which means she will aggravate warm and dry conditions. Christopher Hobbs stated in his book, *Herbal Remedies for Dummies*, that feverfew is the most reliable emmenagogue in the *Materia Medica*.

In the 1980s, studies showed her effectiveness with migraine headaches. A member of the daisy family, she has been used for centuries for headaches, arthritis, and problems with labor and childbirth. Greek physicians used it as an anti-inflammatory and for menstrual cramps. Feverfew is effective for reducing fevers, as her name suggests.

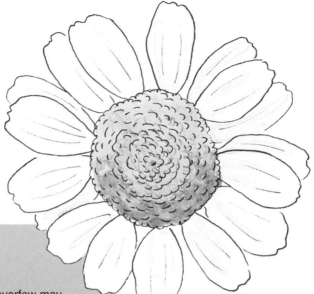

Note

The side effects of feverfew may include abdominal pain, gas, indigestion, diarrhea, nausea, vomiting, and nervousness. If raw leaves are chewed fresh you may experience loss of taste and lip, mouth, and tongue swelling. Feverfew allergies could be present for people who are allergic to chamomile, ragweed, or yarrow. Feverfew increases bleeding if you are on any blood thinners. Do not take if pregnant or give to children under the age of two. Feverfew may interact with anesthesia. Do not stop abruptly if you have been taking feverfew for longer than a week. Instead, gradually reduce the dose to avoid side effects. Know your body, know your herbs.

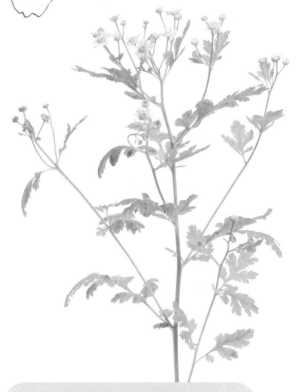

Make

To make an herbal infusion, steep 1 ounce (28 g) feverfew in 2 cups (480 ml) water overnight. Keep covered to capture the volatile oils. In the morning, gently simmer for 40 to 60 minutes to release more minerals. Consume 2 to 4 cups (480 to 940 ml) daily.

Look-alikes

Feverfew is sometimes confused with chamomile.

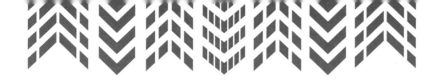

LAVENDER

Lavandula angustifolia

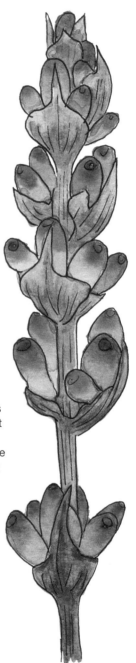

From *lavare*, Latin for "to wash," lavender has a long history and is thought to be grown in the Garden of Eden, possibly one of the oils to anoint Jesus, and used by the Egyptians for mummification. Hildegard of Bingen wrote about lavender in her Latin text to influence the intellects, the clergy, and the political leaders. In her ninth book, *Causes and Cures*, she states that lavender gives "pure knowledge and pure spirit." Hildegard suggested adding lavender flowers to "allay the pains of the liver and the lungs."

Nicholas Culpeper, a maverick seventeenth-century herbalist and considered the father of contemporary alternative medicine, had a clinical herbal practice for the less privileged in London. His greatest contribution was translating the Latin text of the *Pharmacopoeia Londinensis* to demystify medicine. In his writings, he wrote that lavender helped with all griefs, eased pain of the head and brain, strengthened the stomach and spleen, and was good for stomach irritability and anxiety. Her diffusive action influences the outer branches of the nervous system, our restlessness. She is one of the main ingredients for the four thieves vinegar to cleanse the skin. Lavender can help shift our emotional and hormonal states; it helps release excessive anger, let the fire out, chill our spirit, and cheer our heart.

Lavender's fragrance may carry many memories from our childhood. Folks often say she reminds them of their grandmother. Isn't it interesting that she is considered an aphrodisiac? She is another aromatic ally in the mint family that is cultivated for perfumes, soaps, cosmetics, detergents, and aromatherapy. Varieties are natural mutations that can be propagated by seed or cuttings, like *Lavandula angustifolia* var. *munstead*. To propagate, cut the new tender, green shoots and place in water or plant them directly in the soil, keeping it moist to establish the roots.

There are forty-seven known species of *Lavandula* and hundreds of cultivars. She is possibly one of the most modified plants besides corn, with many hybrids and varieties. Hybrids are two different species bred with a greater diversity than their parents, like *Lavandula* x *intermedia* 'Grosso' or 'Provence'. Cultivars are bred with our help to create a plant with certain characteristics, like *Lavandula stoechas* 'Anouk', whose showy purple flowers stand upright with the appearance of rabbit ears, attracting butterflies.

Lavandula angustifolia is able to grow in cooler climates from her native lands of Spain, Bulgaria, Croatia, and Italy, where she is found in the high mountain regions. Sun loving, she prefers dry alkaline soils growing through Zones 5 to 8. Make sure she has good airflow and coverage to avoid fungal infections.

Plants grown in various altitudes produce different essential oil constituents. This combination of constituents affects the aroma, which can range from floral, herbaceous, earth tones to sharper, pungent, camphor notes. *L. angustifolia* has beautiful floral, earth-woody notes, which is sought after for her aromatic healing properties, creating a relaxed, calm state. The more camphor constituents, like what we find in spike lavender, *L. latifolia*, contains higher camphor notes, which is not relaxing for the body, and in high dosages, toxic to the body. This is a small snapshot of the complexity of essential oils and all the confusion when buying lavender.

Lavender's clean aroma symbolizes love, devotion, and purity. And yet she is a shape-shifter. She can be soothing for the mind for some people and irritating for others. Paradoxically, she brings peace and uplifts our spirits from our cloudy, foggy, anxious, and negative thoughts. She helps clear codependency and influences our intellect by asking for clear communication.

In Spain, it is reported that lavender teas are used to treat diabetes and insulin resistance. She is analgesic, antiseptic, expectorant, a nervine, and a vulnerary. Add 10 percent of her to tea blends as she is potent, and her bitter aromatics will overpower the blend. Lavender's polyphenol compounds are a type of antioxidant to reduce "bad" bacteria in the gut from antibiotics. Sprinkle a very small amount of the dried flowers onto Greek yogurt to reduce bloating and improve digestion. Add to vinegars, wine, food, and simple syrups. Create a lavender icing for your lemon cake. The best shortbread I ever made had lavender flowers in the batter. Remember to follow a recipe for amounts as she has a powerful aroma. When applying lavender essential oil directly on the skin, use small amounts for her antimicrobial action.

continued on next page

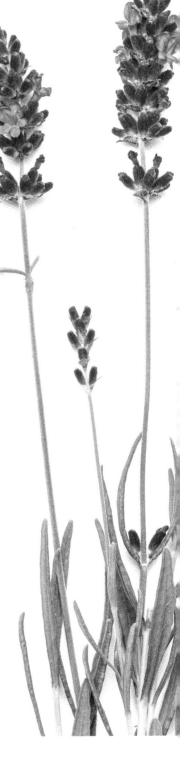

Make

Sip a little lavender tea for your immune system or use the tea as a facial toner. Add 5 tablespoons (70 g) fresh lavender flowers and a 750 ml bottle of red wine to a pot on the stovetop. Bring to a boil and then simmer for 30 to 45 minutes to evaporate the alcohol. Let cool, strain, and rebottle. Take 2 tea-spoons (10 ml) three times daily for 10 days.

For constipation, nervous bellies, or headaches, make an alcohol tincture with both the flower and the leaf in a 1:5 ratio in 70 percent alcohol. Make the tincture with glycerin to use for children. Prepare the herbs as incense, or place whole flowers or powdered herb on charcoal. Add to potpourri, or use as an insect repellent. Steep lavender in tea to use on your scalp as a dandruff rinse.

Musings

As mentioned previously, essential oils are very potent medicines and should be used with great care. When chemical compounds are isolated they have the potential to harm, hence why we want the complete plant to balance out their potency. Do not ingest essential oils.

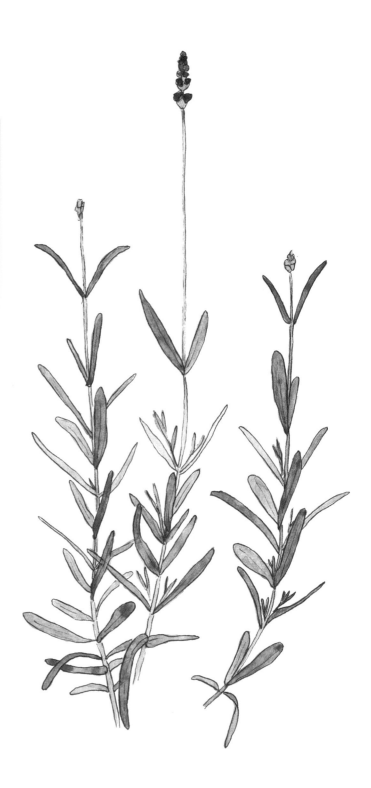

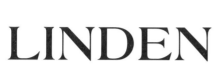

LINDEN

Tilia species

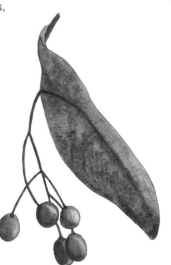

I will always remember my dear friend Alesine, who had asked me where to find linden flowers in the city. I love walking and making note of places where I see plants that I can revisit. When linden flowers are in bloom, there is an abundance of bees buzzing around. Whether they are small or large trees, this food source is like an ocean for our pollinators. Linden stores the warming rays of the sun in her honey sweet blooms, transferring that warmth to our bodies. Cattle love to eat her foliage fresh or dried, so be mindful not to plant out in the pasture.

The fragrant flowers carry volatile oils, tannins, and sugar gums, along with chlorophyll and farnesol, and is an antispasmodic and a sedative. The bark is comprised of tilicin and tiliadin and the leaves are full of saccharine. She contains flavonoids and is a diaphoretic, which helps induce sweating to reduce fevers. Her mucilage soothes bronchitis as she calms the receptors and promotes healing of the airways.

Collect the flowers when they are just opening and infuse for anxiety, nervous vomiting, or palpitations. Use linden to alleviate stuffy noses, clear nasal passages, and break up mucus in the throat. Linden is incredibly soothing for the skin and lovely in a warm bath. Linden flowers are used for blood pressure, insomnia, incontinence, and joint swelling. Use caution with pregnancy, and when using lithium or heart medications.

Make

Blend equal parts linden flowers, yarrow, and St. John's wort for a tea to break up mucus. Drink extra fluids to flush out the kidneys. For a relaxing tea to lessen nervous tension, combine 1 cup (240 ml) hot water, 1.5 ounces (42 g) linden flowers, ⅔ ounce (18 g) sage, ⅔ ounce (18 g) thyme, and ⅔ ounce (18 g) lemon balm. Add honey to sweeten.

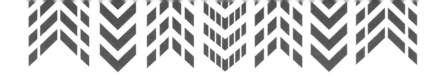

MILK THISTLE

Silybum marianum

I was introduced to milk thistle when she arrived mysteriously in the Medicine Wheel Garden. She needs a lot of room to grow, with her spiky, needle-edged, milk-spotted leaves. Once her flower head turns to seed you must be diligent to collect before her fruit, achene—what we call her seeds—float all over your garden. Wear thick clothing and gloves to avoid being pricked by her extremely sharp spikes.

High temperatures and drier environments increase her medicine. Milk thistle has been in use for over two centuries for liver, kidney, and spleen ailments, jaundice, gall-stones, and menstrual pain. Today, milk thistle is helpful for the treatment of hepatitis and cirrhosis. It can also protect liver cells if someone has mistakenly ingested death cap fungus (*Amanita phalloides*). Milk thistle reduces cytokine storms of inflammation, is an antioxidant, scavenges free radicals, reduces liver fibrosis, and balances blood sugars. Known as a "liver protector," she is a bitter tonic, cholagogue, detoxifier, anti-viral, and antioxidant. Research from Iran is showing promise that milk thistle reduces cancer tumor growth in the liver, pancreas, prostate, and breast. There is conflicting research about taking milk thistle seeds during chemotherapy. Do your research and consult with an herbalist for the best course of action.

Make

As a long-standing edible food in Europe, milk thistle leaves were added to salads, and stalks, roots, and flowers were cooked for various recipes. Eat her crunchy seeds in salads. Make a coffee substitute with her seeds. Her medicine is not water-soluble. Tincture her seeds in alcohol to capture the active ingredient of silymarin; it will make a yellow medicine.

Note

There are a few cautions about milk thistle. She may potentiate diabetes medication. Milk thistle may interact with antipsychotics, birth control pills, hormone replacement therapy, antibiotics, and immunosuppressant and hepatitis medications. Avoid when pregnant and breastfeeding.

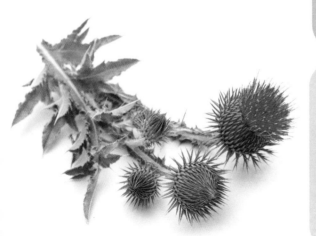

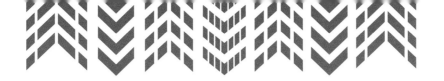

MULLEIN

Verbascum thapsus

I was always happy to witness greater mullein growing tall on barren lands as we traveled through our semidesert area, what is known as British Columbia. A few years ago, she appeared in the landscape of one of the curated gardens here in the city. She is now considered a naturalized plant. Mullein originates from Eurasia and North Africa and arrived here on the shores around the 1700s. In Virginia, she was used as a piscicide to stun the fish for easy fishing. She traveled across the Midwest with new settlers around 1839 and finally arrived on the Pacific Coast in 1876.

The Lenape People of Oklahoma used mullein for cold remedies and as an antirheumatic. The Mi'kmaq Peoples reportedly used it as a respiratory aid and for asthma. It was noted in Moerman's ethnobotany book that the Iroquois made poultices by heating the leaf and applying it directly to the skin for earaches and hemorrhoids. The Zuni powdered the root for their poultices applied on sores and wounds. There are many entries for various Nations and Tribes and their interconnection with this new relative to Turtle Island.

Mullein contains flavonoids, is mucilaginous, and is high in saponins, tannins, and volatile oils. Medicinal actions are as an expectorant for bronchitis, deep thick coughs, and chest colds. You can burn the leaves or dry the leaves and use as a steam inhalant. It's also used as a demulcent, an anti-inflammatory, and an antispasmodic.

Mullein is fuzzy on the top and bottom of the leaf, capturing and directing rainwater down to her root. She is what we refer to as a "people's plant," as most of our "common weeds" are in service and find opportunity for prime real estate on open, sunny spaces. Mullein likes it dry and does not do well in wet soil. She hosts a variety of insects, along with both short- and long-tongued bees. Her flowers are autogamous, so if she is not pollinated, she can self-pollinate at the end of the day. She produces 100,000 to 250,000 viable seeds for decades, possibly centuries, for future mullein plants. The seeds need sunlight for germination, so when we disturb the soil we might be bringing her age-old seeds to the surface.

Harvest the leaves before flowering. You can take the midriff off the leaf to speed the drying process. Do not gather any mullein growing along the highways, as her fuzzy underleaf collects sticky, black gunk. When making tea, be sure to strain the plant material well so you don't drink her irritating, fuzzy leaves.

continued on next page

Make

Once dried, grind her leaves through a sieve for teas. Serve with honey for soothing sore throats. Collect flowers in the morning and place them in a clean jar with oil for an infusion. Place her fresh flowers in water and allow the sunlight to extract her oil, skimming off the mullein oil on top with an eyedropper. Store the oils in the fridge over winter until the following year. Infused mullein oil is very helpful for ear infections, especially with St. John's wort and garlic. Heat the mullein oil and add some fresh minced garlic. Once warm, administer a few drops into the ear, massaging lightly around the earlobes and down the neck. This medicine is not recommended for swimmer's ear or a punctured eardrum.

Note

Mullein contains rotenone, an insecticide, and coumarin, which can prevent blood from clotting. Avoid it if there are any liver or kidney concerns.

Musings

We could collect the seeds and disperse them alongside our roads to absorb the cars' pollutants and keep toxins out of our waterways.

Look-alikes

Mullein can be confused with foxglove (*Digitalis purpurea*), which contains a cardiac glycoside, digitoxin, a powerful and poisonous compound. To tell the difference, look for foxglove's toothed leaves with less hair than mullein's leaf.

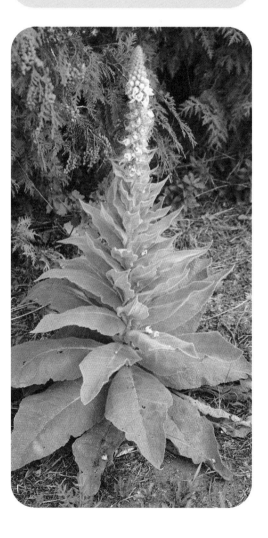

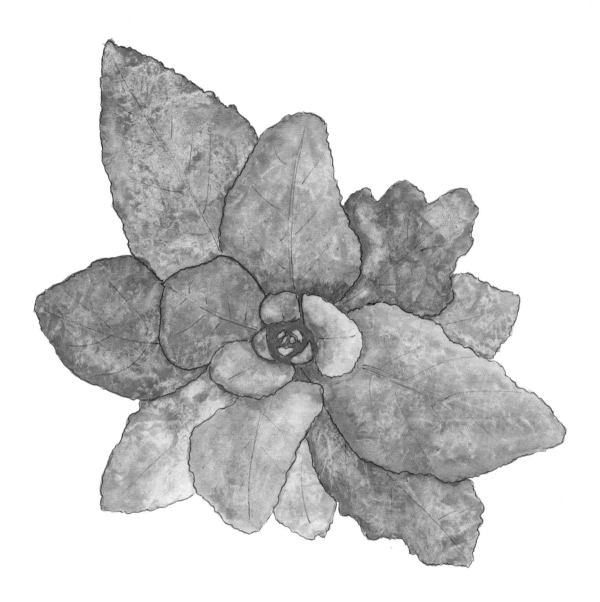

Toby Hemenway's book, *Gaia's Garden*, speaks about our opportunistic Rooted Nations, which flourish in neglected meadows, pastures, vacant lots, industrial sites, and open sunny spaces. Our More-Than-Human-Kin move in to repair and rebuild the humus and fungal layers. Greater mullein harvests the energy of Grandfather Sun to reconstruct the life cycle and reconnect what has been severed. We need those thickets of fast-growing pioneer plants building biomass and homes and food for deer and rabbits. Our plants quickly restitch disturbed sites back together, reweaving them into functioning ecosystems. Mullein is a common weed that provides seeds for our migrating winged kin, including goldfinches (*Spinus tristis*).

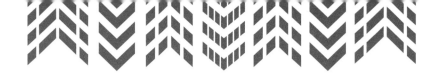

MOTHERWORT

Leonurus cardiaca

I was happy to discover that someone's had "guerrilla gardened" a new guest into the Medicine Wheel Garden: motherwort. It had been a few decades since I first met motherwort and I didn't recognize her until she stabbed me with her pokey calyx! Motherwort grows up to 3 feet (1 m) tall and is a herbaceous perennial in the Lamiaceae family. Her leaves are palmately lobed and covered with stiff hairs. Her little pink flowers are grouped in clusters found at the leaf axil.

Any of our herbs that end with the old Saxon word *wort* refers to the plant as a medicine. Drink motherwort tea and you just may live a long, strong life. Motherwort is a cardiac tonic and an intense nervine, offering her medicine for our heart, our nerves, and our uterus. *Cardiaca* is named specifically for the muscle of the heart and the herb is particularly helpful for genetic conditions. Motherwort stimulates and helps the heart repair itself. She is used for postpartum agitation, PMS, panic attacks, hot flashes, and feeling overwhelmed, especially in mothers.

Her tea is very bitter, but you can mask the flavor with other mints or infuse it with honey. Collect the top third of her just as she blooms around summer solstice. Antibacterial, antioxidant, and anti-inflammatory, she has been adopted by many Tribes and Nations for gastrointestinal issues and "female ills" and as a sedative. Note she is considered invasive in some areas around Turtle Island, possibly a medicine for those folks who are pulling her out!

Musings

I pray over my medicine, in particular when it is so bitter and I have noticed that my body receives her with a deeper appreciation.

Make

Steep 1 teaspoon motherwort in 1 cup (240 ml) boiling water and drink two or three times daily. Dry and powder motherwort to fill capsules. Although the bioactive compounds are water-soluble and best released in a water infusion, decoction, or alcohol tincture, the capsules are more palatable. Make a strong medicine for serious conditions, but if you drink more than 4 cups (960 ml) you will probably feel quite sedated.

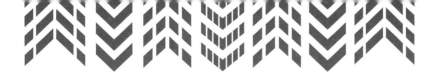

OREGON GRAPE

Berberis aquifolium
Berberis nervosa

Oregon grape, *Berberis aquifolium*, grows in colonies in moist soil and is a great hedgerow plant. *B. aquifolium* grows tall, offering a good prickly, protective fence. She was prepared by North American Tribes and Nations for various ailments like stomach complaints, arthritis, tuberculosis, and syphilis, and for natural dyes and food. Around 1824, the Scottish botanist David Douglas visited Turtle Island, identifying and classifying our native plants into the Latin system of naming. Employed as a botanical collector with the Royal Horticultural Society of London, he introduced Oregon grape to the English countryside, and it now grows predominantly in Brighton on the coast of England. These plants in the *Mahonia* genus were recently moved to *Berberis*.

B. aquifolium, a broadleaf leathery evergreen shrub, grows up to 10 feet (3 m) tall by 5 feet (1.5 m) wide. *B. nervosa* grows much lower to the ground with upright flowering stalks. Oregon grape blooms April to May with bright clusters of canary yellow flowers, which are edible. After pollination, her very sour, dark blue-purplish berries can be collected and mixed with other wild berries to make fruit leather, syrup, wine, or jam. Her compound leaf with various numbers of leaflets are opposite on a woody stem and turn red in the fall, when they decrease in chlorophyll. The young leaves are foraged for side garnishes and for the floral industry. Oregon grape can be propagated by seeds. She is slow to start, but once established will easily naturalize.

Collect her roots and bark any time of the year. As the roots grow horizontally, she produces many clones. You can dig up a portion of the root, around 12 inches (30 cm), without taking her life. The bark contains the beneficial compound berberine, along with the alkaloids berbamine and palmatine, which support a synergistic effect when using the whole plant. Berberine is also found in goldenseal (*Hydrastis canadensis*). It is an active constituent that contains a strong MDR inhibitor, 5'-methoxyhydnocarpin. Berberine demonstrates a strong resistance to methicillin-resistant *Staphylococcus aureus*, known as MRSA. Oregon grape is helpful for diarrhea, lowers blood sugars, modulates inflammation, alleviates parasitic infections caused by bacteria, treats skin issues, and soothes dry, red,

continued on next page

teary eyes. The bark is used medicinally for stagnant liver, gallbladder disorders, poor digestion, urinary tract infections, skin issues, and macular degeneration.

The bitter flavor of Oregon grape root activates the gastrointestinal tract. Her flavor stimulates saliva, which turns on a cascade of digestive functions, such as stimulating the liver and gallbladder for bile, digestive enzymes, and the hydro-chloric acids that break down our food. Bitters are cooling, help drain a sluggish liver, and activate peristalsis, moving the bile into the bowels. With the stimula-tion of the liver and gallbladder activating the detoxification process, be mindful of its possible interaction with birth control pills, thyroid medicine, and heart medications. This process will flush medications more quickly out of your body.

Oregon grape offers many gifts to a diversity of insects who visit her. When we observe our Relatives and the community they live in, we create healthy relations.

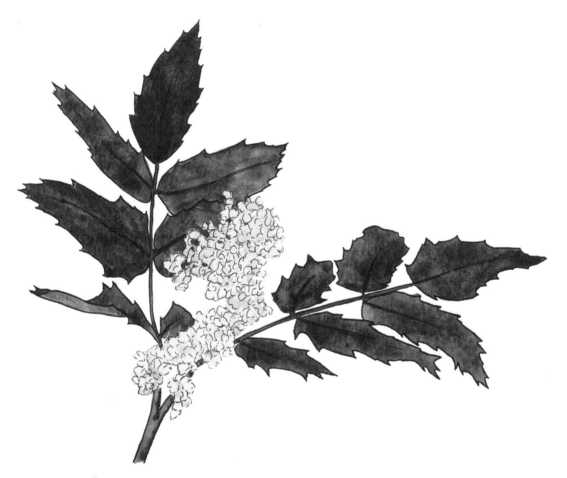

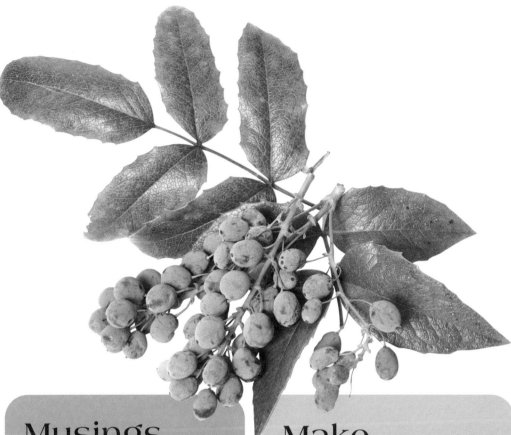

Musings

With hedgerows or guilds, a community of diverse Relatives who grow together, collaborating and co-creating a living barrier with a variety of diverse More-Than-Human-Kin. We can avoid metal and wooden fences and create habitat.

There is a difference between wild-crafters and extractors (those only concerned with making a profit). Check out United Plant Savers to know what plants in your area may be on the threatened or endangered lists. Check in with your local Nation or Tribe, forge a relationship, and see if they might have plants you are looking to reintroduce and tend.

Make

Use Oregon grape in teas, tinctures, infused oils, dusting powder for wounds, and salves. Steep a tea for mouthwash to treat a sore throat. Combine the berries with other berry types and turn them into fruit leather, syrup, wine, or jam. Michael Moore's book, *Medicinal Plants of the Mountain West*, states that Oregon grape is helpful for symptoms of an adrenal junkie, constipation with dry skin, and a coated tongue in the morning. He recommends 30 to 45 drops of tincture three times daily for at least 2 weeks.

To be in right relationship with yourself is the biggest gift you can give yourself. Check in with your lifestyle. Meditate, exercise, eat a healthy diet, and sleep well.

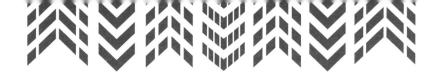

STRAWBERRY

Fragaria chiloensis
Fragaria vesca
Fragaria virginiana

Strawberry is known as the heart berry—the fruit of the womb—symbolizing fertility and sacred renewal. She helps us understand connection to the four directions, one of our Indigenous teachings that helps us balance our mental, emotional, physical, and spiritual. All over the globe many cultures hold teachings, guidance, and annual feasts honoring the changing season. We need our heart to guide us, as love is an alive, dynamic experience, an action of commitment, compassion, and caring.

Today we find strawberry cultivated worldwide. As we regain our roots, we regain the stories that go back to France around 1300 CE, here on Turtle Island, and to South America, where strawberries were traded. In Asia around 2600 BCE, the Yellow Emperor drank tea made of strawberry leaves for detoxifying and reducing the effects of aging. During the Roman Empire, strawberry was shared to lift spirits, for digestive complaints, and to alleviate bad breath. As a member of the rose family, strawberries carry love. I am reminded that there are many Indigenous teachings about strawberry. I share with the children that the leaf helps us let go of anger and the fruit helps us forgive. Let's contemplate the gift of strawberry with seasonal eating, to be mindful how she is grown, create balance, and practice reciprocal relationships.

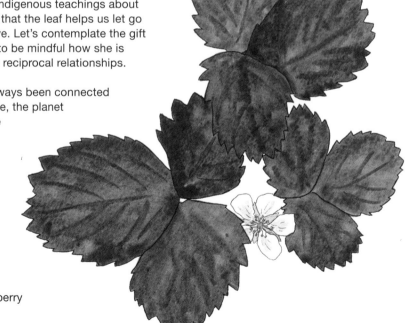

In our European mythos, she has always been connected with the goddesses Freyja, Aphrodite, the planet Venus, and the Virgin Mary. To share the fruit of strawberry with another will bring love. My Anishinaabe ancestors refer to her as *o-day'min*, whose seeds are on the outside, representing us, teaching about our vulner-ability. The Haudenosaunee speak of strawberry as the symbol of life and health. They would dry the fruit to make leather strips. The Oneida People mashed strawberry with corn to make strawberry

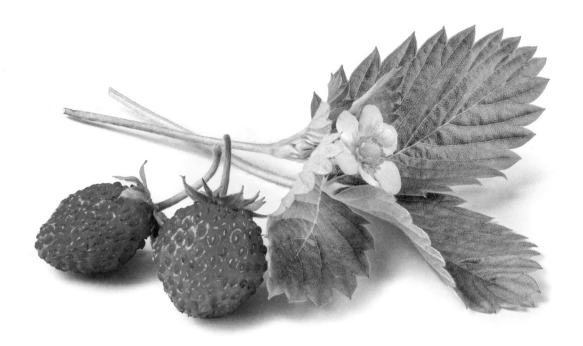

bread. They also made medicine with the root and leaf to treat diarrhea, inflammation, and achy joints.

During the 1800s, in the greenhouse of the royal palace in Versailles, they cultivated our American strawberry (*Fragaria virginiana*) with Chilean strawberry (*Fragaria chiloensis*), creating a hybrid, *Fragaria* x *ananassa*. *Ananassa* means "pineapple" in French and invokes her large, sweet, aggregate fruit.

Today, strawberries grow year-round in the state of California, producing 20,000 pounds (9,100 kg) per acre (0.4 ha) based on farming practices. To overcome the disease of Verticillium wilt, the industrial farms use chloropicrin, the tear gas that was produced during the First World War. Once strawberries are harvested, they will not produce any more sugar. In regenerative farming practices, the yield will be smaller, at 5,000 pounds (2,300 kg) per acre (0.4 ha), and the fruit is picked when ripe and full of medicine.

Flowering from March to May, strawberry is easy to grow in full sun to partial shade in rich, moist, well-drained soil. Mulch with straw and ensure good airflow to protect from disease. Strawberry attracts many pollinators, such as Sara orangetip butterflies and our Winged Relatives such as robins, waxwings, and towhees. She is the host plant for checkerspot butterfly larvae. Snip off the first flower to stimulate more flower growth. The flower has both male (stamen) and female (pistil) organs, which is pollinated to become an achene.

continued on next page

The swollen receptacle becomes full with over two hundred achene, the outside seeds. The baby runners will detract from growing berries as the energy is going into growing a new plant. Snip off runners to stimulate fruit growth. You can place the runners in water to grow roots and create more ground cover or give away to your neighbors.

The berries are full of phytonutrients, flavonoids, anthocyanins, and ellagic acid, which is considered an anticarcinogenic. It may actively treat cancers of the breast, esophagus, skin, colon, prostate, and pancreas. She is also rich in calcium, copper, fiber, folate, iodine, iron, magnesium, manganese, omega-3s, potassium, and vitamins A, B2, B5, B6, C, and K. Strawberry helps reduce inflammation, pulling heat out of irritated skin like acne and sunburn, and may help with scarring. Harvest the astringent leaf before the flower; it is high in vitamin C and iron. Strawberry tea has been reported to regulate menstruation, calm morning sickness, help with breast milk production, and is a mild nerve tonic.

Make

Mix the fresh berries with baking soda to help whiten your teeth, as the malic acid is a natural whitener. Make an exfoliating face mask with a handful of fresh berries, the juice of 1 lemon, and ½ cup (120 g) yogurt. Blend together, chill for 20 minutes, then apply to the face and neck. Make a tea for facial steams to reduce oily skin or make a fresh berry tea toner.

Musings

When making teas, make sure the herb is completely fresh for mild, light teas or completely dry for capturing their intense flavor.

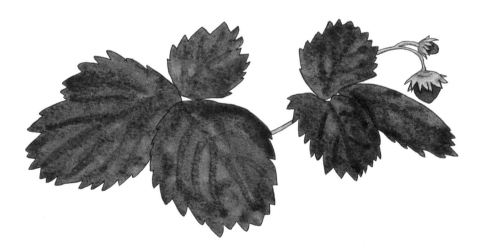

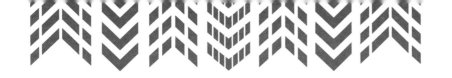

ST. JOHN'S WORT

Hypericum perforatum

Back in the 1800s, if your neighbor was sad, overwhelmed, and anxious (not unlike many of us are today), you would have thought they were possessed. The village herbalist would recommend they drink St. John's wort tea and after several weeks the neighbor would report that they felt like a light inside them had turned back on. That's because this magical healing plant is said to aid with mild to moderate depression. Research in Germany officially recognized St. John's wort to be helpful for depression in 1984.

St. John's wort is often labeled a weed, which doesn't represent her true attributes. Perhaps this reference comes from her growing in pastures where cattle might be affected by her medicines. Like so many "weeds," there can be a lot of conflicting information and we sometimes forget how long these medicinal healing herbals have been growing around us, offering their lives so we can live ours.

St. John's wort is described as a midsize perennial with yellow flowers. What differentiates them from others in the *Hypericum* genus are the "perforations" in the leaf, filled with red resinous glands of hypericin and other active compounds. St. John's wort spreads by seed as well as by an active vegetative root. It will grow up to 3 feet (91 cm) tall by 2 feet (61 cm) wide in USDA plant hardiness Zones 5 through 10. St. John's wort grows well in sand, clay, rocky soil, or loam, and tolerates an acidic to slightly alkaline pH. She can grow in semi-shade (light woodland) or no shade and moist soil. She flowers from May to August, and the seeds ripen from July to September.

The species is hermaphrodite (has both male and female organs) and is pollinated by bees and flies. The plant is self-fertile. According to the Invasive Species Alert in the United States and Canada, St. John's wort is often considered a noxious weed and is also referred to as Klamath weed. The BC Invasive Species Council warns that St. John's wort can cause injury to light-skinned cattle. She has a protective covering on her seeds that allows her to survive for up to ten years, and a single plant can produce up to 100,000 seeds.

continued on next page

Collect St. John's wort from June to late August. She is found anywhere the soil has been disturbed: open woods, grasslands, in dry sunny places, along roadways, in the cracks of sidewalks, alongside pastures, or even in your garden. You can identify St. John's wort by holding the leaf up to the light to look for the small glands that look like holes. There are ten times more glands in the flower than the leaf or stem, which is why the flower is so often used in herbalism. The best time to gather her is in the midday when the medicine is at its height. Harvest the flower tops, leaf, and stem. The stems are quite stiff, so use scissors.

St. John's wort healing properties are due to the presence of hypericin, which is known to interfere with monoamine oxidase (MOA), which contributes to depression. Pharmaceutical products also act as MOA inhibitors; however, St. John's wort is slower acting and has few side effects. Here in the Pacific Northwest we can have long, cloudy winters with little sun, so I use her daily as my facial moisturizer. She repairs tissue damage and is very effective for seasonal affective disorder (SAD). Some people who are fair-skinned report that they are more sensitive to the sun when using St. John's wort oil; however, the sun is not as strong in the winter.

St. John's wort is also used for the digestive and nervous systems. It improves the absorption of nutrients and normalizes stomach acid levels, which fluctuate as we age. She is also helpful for ulcers, heartburn, bloating, bedwetting, menstrual challenges, menopause, and liver tension, as it gently decongests and strengthens the liver and the gallbladder. A research paper in 2000 raised a new concern. St. John's wort extract was shown to improve liver function. Although this would normally be considered a good thing, this paper raised the concern that improved liver function might cause pharmaceutical drugs to be broken down more quickly and could mean that people who needed to have a drug active in their system twenty-four hours per day could now in theory have a gap where the drug was not active.

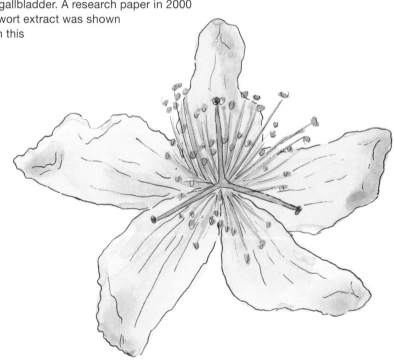

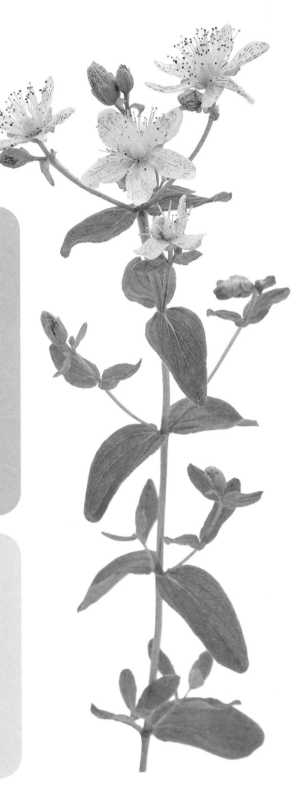

Make

This herb, with her flowers and leaves, needs to be fresh when infusing into oils. Place the oil in the sun until she turns bright red, usually within a month. Apply to the skin for back pain, sciatica, neuralgia, arthritic joints, wounds, surgical scars, bruises, and sprains. Make an alcohol tincture for seasonal affective disorder, liver congestion, shingles, nervous exhaustion, menopausal moods, viral infections, and jet lag. Start with ¼ to 1 teaspoon three times a day. Notice how you react and adjust the dosage for your body type.

Note

It's best not to use St. John's wort when taking contraceptives or pharmaceuticals. Do not take St. John's wort with antidepressants without the supervision of an herbalist or medical practitioner. As with any herb, it is important that you do your research and check with your health care professional before using it, as it may have interactions with other medications.

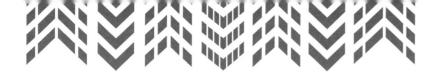

UVA URSI

Arctostaphylos uva-ursi

Uva ursi, also known as bearberry or kinnikinnick, creeps as an evergreen mat over bare rocks, lying low, covering Mother Earth. Latin for "grape of the bear," she reminds us that whatever bear eats, we can eat. In the late fall, bears clean out their intestines from tapeworms and parasites by eating uva ursi berries. They follow this by chewing on rough-edged sedge, which helps drag out pathogens. The berries are a carbohydrate, high in vitamin C, and a powerful antimicrobial.

A dear friend has a wild patch on the property where she lives. I was grateful to have the chance to taste her flavorful, bright red berry because the other places I have tasted her gift were not as sweet. I was reminded that our More-Than-Human-Kin are in relationship with their environment: the altitude, the quality of the soil, and the love we offer, all of which bring sweetness to the fruit.

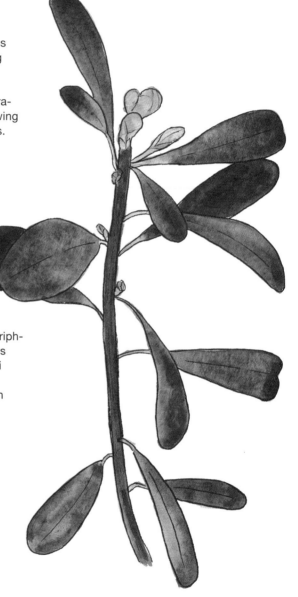

Gather her leaves in late summer, collecting from the periphery of the mat. Make sure there are no black fungal spots on her leaf to be infused in tinctures or for teas. Uva ursi is excellent for mouth infections, diarrhea, cystitis, and nephritis. One of the chemical compounds, arbutin, is an antiseptic that converts to hydroquinone. For the hydroquinone to be effective, we need our inner environment to be alkaline. Dissolve 1 teaspoon of baking soda in water and drink the mixture 30 minutes before taking the medicine. To activate the arbutin, it must be absorbed intact through the intestine to the urinary system. When we isolate and take synthetic medications, the bacteria in the intestine will break it down before it has a chance to be absorbed for its effectiveness. This is why whole plant medicine works best. There are many chemical constituents that are working together in ways we have not yet discovered.

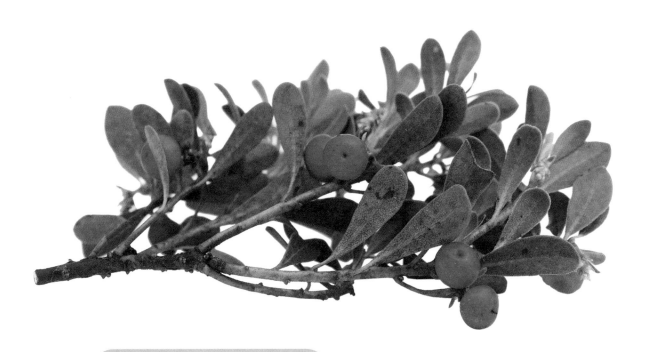

Make

Steep an overnight cold water infusion with crushed leaves, which contain fewer tannins and more arbutin. Drink 1 cup (240 ml) of the infusion three times a day. For tinctures, take 10 drops three times a day until symptoms dissipate. You may notice your urine is a light green in color, which is harmless.

Note

It's best to avoid uva ursi when pregnant. Also, raw berries in large quantities can be toxic or cause constipation.

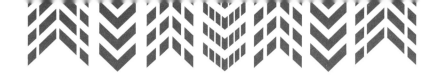

SASKATOON BERRY

Amelanchier alnifolia

I had the pleasure to first meet saskatoon berry when I traveled into the interior of British Columbia to visit one of my herb girlfriends. She is sometimes known as service-berry, juneberry, alder-leaf shad berry, or shadberry. With pome fruit that looks similar to blueberries, I was invited to taste and was instantly enamored with her sweet, tangy flavor with hints of nutty almond.

Her Cree name is *mis-ask-quah-toomina*, meaning "fruit of the tree with many branches." Saskatoon berry has a long history and tradition with numerous Tribes and Nations here on Turtle Island. The Blackfoot harvested the dark brown to grayish, hard wood that was relatively straight for arrows, pipes, and tipi closure pins. The juice of the berries was applied as eardrops or an eyewash for sore eyes. The berries were dried in the sun and mixed with various meats, like buffalo, deer, or moose, and animal fats to make pemmican, which could be stored for long periods of time. Teas were made with the leaves, twigs, and roots to be used for upset stomach, constipation, menstruation, miscarriage, childbirth recovery, and contraception. When saskatoon berries ripen around the summer solstice, it marks a time to gather with other Tribes, where saskatoon berries are traded for sacred tobacco. Small ceremonial prairie plots were dug and plant-ed with berries, elk manure, and seeds to grow tobacco.

In his book *Plants and the Blackfoot*, Alex Johnston wrote that the Blackfoot used saska-toon for the treatment and prevention of diabetes. The National Library of Medicine pub-lished a paper with grant funding from Diabetes Canada to explore her medicinal prop-erties in animal testing. Some basic research has clarified certain functions. Saskatoon berry strongly inhibits aldose reductase, which is closely related to diabetic complications such as cataracts, neuropathy, kidney disease, retinopathy, and atherosclerosis. The phenolic acids, anthocyanins, and proanthocyanidins lower blood sugar levels. Saska-toon berry leaf extract potently suppresses mammalian α-glucosidase activity and delays the absorption of carbohydrates, significantly lowering blood glucose. Polyphenols can also reduce blood glucose levels. Saskatoon berry is therefore an alternative medicine for preventing and treating diabetes.

 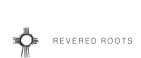

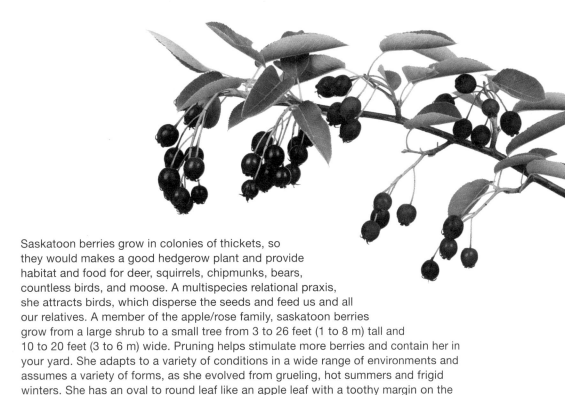

Saskatoon berries grow in colonies of thickets, so they would makes a good hedgerow plant and provide habitat and food for deer, squirrels, chipmunks, bears, countless birds, and moose. A multispecies relational praxis, she attracts birds, which disperse the seeds and feed us and all our relatives. A member of the apple/rose family, saskatoon berries grow from a large shrub to a small tree from 3 to 26 feet (1 to 8 m) tall and 10 to 20 feet (3 to 6 m) wide. Pruning helps stimulate more berries and contain her in your yard. She adapts to a variety of conditions in a wide range of environments and assumes a variety of forms, as she evolved from grueling, hot summers and frigid winters. She has an oval to round leaf like an apple leaf with a toothy margin on the upper part of the leaf. Her wild, white, five-petaled flower can be easily spotted in the spring as she covers almost the entire tree with blooms. Saskatoon berries need full sun and can be susceptible to saskatoon-juniper rust if grown within 1.2 miles (2 km) of juniper. She prefers moist, well-drained soil. Since her root system is shallow, it's best not to grow grass under her branches. Keep her well mulched without touching the base of her trunk.

Saskatoon berry contains twenty-six essential nutrients, vitamin C, and antioxidants. She increases our energy, improves stamina and vitality, boosts the immune system, reduces inflammation, balances blood sugar, and lowers cholesterol. Our stomachs feel fuller for longer with her 3 grams of fiber per 3.5 ounces (100 g) of fruit, even though she has only 66 calories.

Three cultivars of Saskatoon berries, 'Thiessen', 'Nelson', and 'Smokey' express high radical scavenging activity. *Mis-ask-quah-toomina* brings us back to how the Rooted Nations teach us to be in good relations so that they will take care of us when we take care of them and the land. A reciprocal interconnected relationship of give and take.

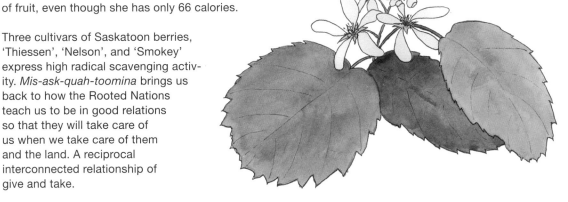

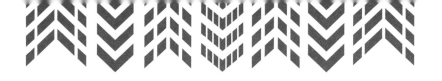

PEARLY EVERLASTING

Anaphalis margaritacea

As a child I would pretend that small rocks were potatoes, little pieces of wood were meat, vine maple leaves were bread, and pearly everlasting was popcorn. I adore this little creamy, papery flower that grows wild in my memories from long ago. Slowly we are seeing her reintroduced to gardens as she is a nectar and host plant for American lady (*Vanessa virginiensis*) and painted lady (*Vanessa cardui*) butterflies. With the butterflies laying their eggs in late April and May, and caterpillars feasting on the leaf, your plants with not look great, but there is still time for her to flower later in the season.

The flower and leaf are used to help dry out extra fluid when the body is congested; she shrinks tissue like a sponge, mopping up the water. Pearly everlasting is helpful for treating hemorrhoids and varicose veins. During the flu epidemic of 1941 in the Carolinas, a pearly everlasting tea with whiskey and lemon was a popular treatment. She is astringent, a mild expectorant, a sedative, and antiseptic. Her fresh juice has been used as an aphrodisiac. During the 1700s and 1800s, her delicate soothing aroma, similar to hops (*Humulus lupulus*), was made into calming pillows.

The Cherokee steamed the leaves to inhale for headaches. The Cheyenne powdered the flowers to rub on the horses' hooves to make them long winded for strong endurance. The Mohegan infused the plant as a cold remedy, and the Haudenosaunee made medicine with the roots and stalks for diarrhea and dysentery. For ceremonial practices, the leaves were burned as incense to purify offerings to Grandfather Sun or to the Spirits.

Pearly everlasting commonly pop up in dry, stony clay soils of mountain meadows, prairies, fallow fields, and disturbed areas. In full sun, we find her all around Turtle Island. Collect pearly everlasting flowers in the late summer. Growing in Zones 3 to 8, she reaches up to 3 feet (91 cm) tall and 2 feet (61 cm) across, with globe-like, pearl white involucre bracts that surround yellow disk flowers. She has

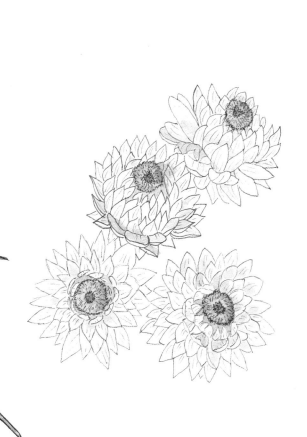

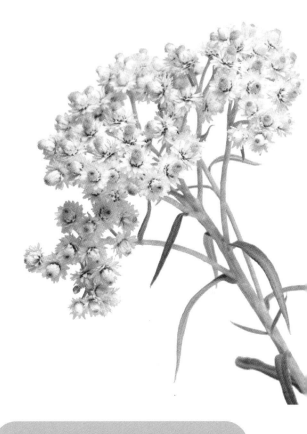

single-sexed flowers, with pistillate yellow centers on one and staminate flowers on the other. You can identify the females by the brown circle around the fragrant tiny yellow pea-size flowers that bloom from July to October. The bracted flowers hold their shape for a long time and have been arranged in floral bouquets for centuries.

Tea made with pearly everlasting releases her bitter, sweet flavor with a licorice aroma and spicy-sweet undertones. The tea can be used for mouthwash, as a mild antihistamine, to reduce edema, and to treat stomach flu. Pearly everlasting offers dyes ranging in tones from green and brown. Apply the fresh herb externally as a poultice for bruising and sunburns.

Make

Harvest the young leaves for wild salads.

Look-alikes

Field balsam or cudweed (*Gnaphalium* ssp.) can be mistaken for pearly everlasting. Field balsam is less fuzzy and smells piney, with the same usages as pearly everlasting but with greater expectorant effects. Both herbs are listed in the *King's American Dispensatory* written by John Uri Lloyd back in 1854.

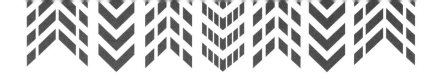

BLACKBERRY

Rubus species

Our native Blackberry (*Rubus ursinus*) here on the West Coast, unfortunately, is crowded out by other introduced species. The evergreen or cut leaf blackberry (*Rubus laciniatus*) is from Eurasia, and the Himalayan blackberry *(Rubus armeniacus)* is a hardy introduced species from Armenia and northern Iran. The evergreen blackberry was planted here with seeds from India in 1885. I rarely refer to introduced species as invasive because I see all our Rooted Nations as teachers. Yet I ask myself, "What do the introduced Kin ask us to pay attention to?" What I have observed is her tenacity.

It was interesting to read that the Himalayan fleshy growing canes contain an anti-feedant compound, 2-heptanol and methyl salicylate. These compounds antagonize insects' neurons to induce feeding deterrence. Banana slugs and aphids are given a strong message to stay away. It makes me wonder whether we could make biopesticides with the cane tips. Many have learned that glyphosate herbicides are futile, fruitless, ineffective, worthless, and feeble attempts to quiet her. Research states that the fruit can contain low quantities of glyphosate one year after treatment and trace amounts can be found twelve years after application. The climate can influence the duration of glyphosate found in plant tissues, mainly in the roots. It is a good reminder to get to know the history of the site before you collect our More-Than-Human-Kin for food and medicine.

The Himalayan blackberry's root system grows deep into Mother Earth and the canes are able to hold water and act like a water reservoir. She asks us to be present and have our hands in the soil. To assist her to be a good guest, make sure she does not crowd out native plants.

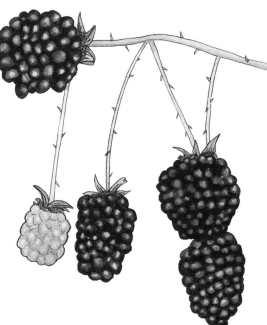

The cane's outer skin can be carefully removed and woven into baskets. Her roots can be used for dyeing fabrics or hair. Medicine is found in the leaf and root bark, which contains antibacterial flavonoids, salicylic acid, and myricetin. She creates a thicket habitat for our Winged Kin, rabbits, and other Relatives, but can easily spread. Cut her back regularly, as the dead canes are fuel for wildfires. Collect the gift of her small aggregate fruit, known as a drupelet, from July to September. The sour flavor reminds us that they are full of vitamin C and phytochemicals like ellagic acid, while the dark fruit's color indicates anthocyanins and polyphenols. Food is the medicine.

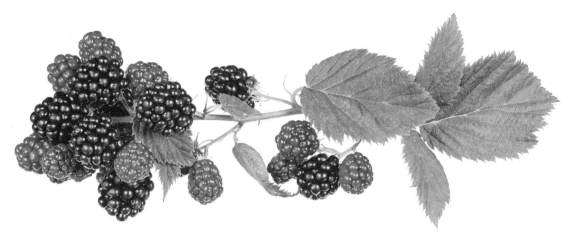

Our First Nations and Native American folk from the Haudenosaunee, Menominee, and Cherokee among many Nations have been developing a highly complex knowledge and oral pharmacopeia. They have been communicating, exchanging knowledge, observing, and practicing with our Rooted Nations for a long time. *Rubus ursinus, R. andrewsianus, R. aliceae*, and *R. trux* are a few of our natives occupying diverse landscapes from acrid to damp conditions; they adapt easily to low or direct sunlight and their seed coats are durable, helping with dispersal from birds. When we have our native blackberry growing more prevalently, then we can all enjoy the local richness that has been co-evolving on Turtle Island for over 20,000 years.

Make

For a topical skin care application that is helpful to rid bacteria growing on the face, like acne, make a tea with dried leaves collected in the fall when the leaf is red. Steep root bark tea for diarrhea, excessive menstruation, fevers, hemorrhoids, sores in the mouth, or urinary tract infections. Harvest the fruit to eat fresh, dehydrate or freeze them. Create sauces, jams, jellies, cordials, and pies.

Musings

Our hands are amazing tools, connecting to the brain and help with our mental health.

ALOE VERA

Aloe vera

Aloe vera is a spiky, cactus-like succulent from the Middle East and is grown worldwide. The word *aloe* is originally from the Arabic word for "shining bitter substance" and *vera* comes from the Latin word "true." Aloe vera is an ancient remedy that was first recorded on clay tablets in Sumerian hieroglyphics during the Mesopotamian era around 2200 BCE. She has been documented in Egypt, Greece, and China as a laxative. During the seventeenth century, she was cultivated by the Spanish in the Caribbean to be sold in Europe. In the 1920s, the United States began growing aloe vera in Florida. We can easily grow her in pots and invite her into our homes.

She is classified as a strong laxative according to David Hoffmann's book, *Medical Herbalism: The Science and Practice of Herbal Medicine*. The presence of anthraquinones—aloin is found in her skin and emodin in her gel—stimulates peristalsis action in the bowels, moving waste out of the body. This also has a similar effect on the uterus. This constituent is found in other species like *Aloe ferox* and *Aloe perryi* as well. She is soothing, moisturizing, and cooling and helps us adopt natural, healthy, healing ways to live in harmony with nature.

Aloe vera contains eighteen amino acids to boost alkalinity in the body. She also contains several enzymes that break down sugars and fats, and can help relieve inflammation from irritable bowel syndrome and ulcerative colitis. Aloe vera contains over two hundred different compounds, including zinc, copper, selenium, calcium, and vitamins A, B12, C, and E. She also contains monosaccharide and polysaccharide sugar molecules, the fatty acids lupeol and campesterol, the plant hormones auxin and gibberellin, salicylic acid, lignins, and saponins. It's important to note that the saponins help with detoxification and therefore can affect the absorption of some medications. Her polysaturated and monosaturated compounds boost white blood cells to support the immune system. As a mouthwash, she helps with dental plaque, cavity disinfecting, and gingivitis.

The colorless mucilaginous gel has been used extensively for pharmacological and cosmetic applications and in the health food industry. Historically, aloe vera has been applied to burns, insect bites, eczema, and other skin problems for her anti-inflammatory properties. Her gel reduces swelling and pain, promotes wound healing, and neutralizes the destruction of UV rays.

Aloe vera's fleshy leaf contains a clear pulp and two major liquids: a bitter yellow latex with anthraquinone compounds and a clear mucilaginous gel. Scientific research and other literature is laden with inconsistent reporting on aloe vera products. Specifically, the ambiguous term *aloe juice* could refer to the

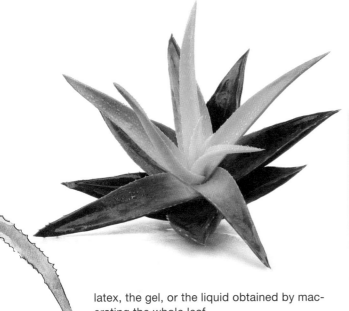

latex, the gel, or the liquid obtained by macerating the whole leaf.

Aloe vera grows thicker, juicier leaves than *Aloe arborescens*, which grows a more stalk-like base, with a thinner, thornier leaf edge. You can grow either species outdoors when it is warm or indoors in a sunny location in well-drained soil. Allow her to dry out between waterings.

Note

If you have allergies to latex, aloe vera may not be your ally. Not everyone can apply or ingest aloe vera. You can skin test it by applying a small amount on the inner arm and waiting twenty-four hours. Some people find it is upsetting and crampy for the stomach. You may need a carminative like peppermint, cardamom, fennel, or ginger when ingesting aloe vera. It is not recommended to ingest aloe vera when pregnant or breastfeeding, for children under the age of twelve, or for anyone with diarrhea. She can be irritating to the stomach and unsafe in large doses.

Make

Mix equal parts coconut oil and sugar, then mix with half the amount of aloe vera and use as an exfoliant once a week or less. Apply daily as a moisturizer, dab on pimples and blackheads, and use as a wash for healthy hair and scalp. She is also known to treat dandruff, so apply aloe vera gel to the scalp, leave on for 30 minutes, and then wash off. Aloe vera helps repair sun-damaged skin cells and reduces the appearance of fine lines and wrinkles. Cut a small ½-inch (1.3 cm) section, slit it lengthwise to expose her pulp, and apply it directly to the skin. I use my nails or a small knife to keep slicing into the gel to receive her goodness. To stabilize the healthy bacteria in your gut, drink 8 ounces (240 ml) before or immediately after a large meal, as to increase the water content in your intestines.

Aloe vera's antibacterial properties help reduce the frequency of acne, psoriasis, and dermatitis. Apply overnight to remove the bacteria and wash up in the morning. Here are some ways to apply it.

● Mix an 8:1 ratio of aloe vera to lemon juice. Blend together, apply, and leave on for 10 minutes, then shampoo off.

● Mix 1 tablespoon (15 ml) aloe vera with 2 tablespoons (30 ml) honey and ¼ teaspoon ground cinnamon. Blend together, apply, and leave on for 10 minutes, then wash off.

● Make a spray with a 2:1 ratio of aloe vera to water.

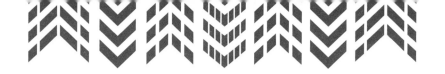

BONESET

Eupatorium perfoliatum

Many Nations and Tribes revered boneset as a really good, effective medicine and our Indigenous relatives shared this knowledge with the first settlers many centuries ago. This knowledge was adopted into the American pharmacopeia in 1892 and today boneset is the only herb to be used by doctors of every school: allopathic, eclectic, and homeopathic. The Alnombak People engaged in the fur trade with European settlers, exchanging their knowledge of boneset to mend bones for knives, fishhooks, and cloth. It was a mutual friendship until the Alnombak People were forced from their homelands.

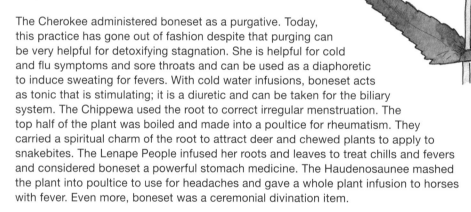

The Cherokee administered boneset as a purgative. Today, this practice has gone out of fashion despite that purging can be very helpful for detoxifying stagnation. She is helpful for cold and flu symptoms and sore throats and can be used as a diaphoretic to induce sweating for fevers. With cold water infusions, boneset acts as tonic that is stimulating; it is a diuretic and can be taken for the biliary system. The Chippewa used the root to correct irregular menstruation. The top half of the plant was boiled and made into a poultice for rheumatism. They carried a spiritual charm of the root to attract deer and chewed plants to apply to snakebites. The Lenape People infused her roots and leaves to treat chills and fevers and considered boneset a powerful stomach medicine. The Haudenosaunee mashed the plant into poultice to use for headaches and gave a whole plant infusion to horses with fever. Even more, boneset was a ceremonial divination item.

A research chemist who specializes in herbal chemistry, Mark Pedersen remarks that boneset is quite versatile. There is not simply one phytochemical, but rather a symbiosis of many constituents that make boneset so powerful for inflammation and infection. Boneset strengthens the immune system by supporting the secretion of interferon, a protein in the family of cytokines. These cytokine molecules communicate to the cells to trigger defense and help eradicate pathogens. Her immunostimulating properties alleviate symptoms of colds and flu and she is an excellent expectorant to loosen phlegm and reduce respiratory inflammation. During the influenza epidemic of 1918/19, boneset set was blended with elderflower with success for the N1H1 virus.

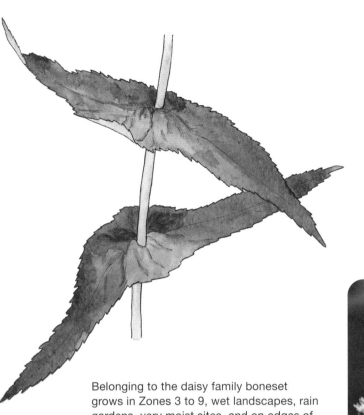

Belonging to the daisy family boneset grows in Zones 3 to 9, wet landscapes, rain gardens, very moist sites, and on edges of swamps with full sun. She grows upward of 2 to 5 feet (61 cm to 1.5 m), and her white flowers and leaves are collected just as she starts to bloom from July to October. As a late season pollinator plant, she is host to thirty-two different species of moths and her stems are nesting sites. Leave the stems standing over winter. Loved by honeybees for the flowers with seeds adored by the birds, boneset has a very bitter taste that is a deterrent for deer and rabbits.

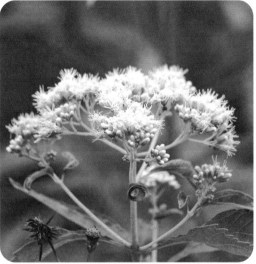

Make

● Make winter cold and flu medicines.

● Make a fresh, finely cut alcohol tincture or a freshly dried chopped tincture. Use in small amounts.

Note

Do not use when pregnant or breast-feeding. Do not use on a long-term basis, as the pyrrolizidine alkaloids can be toxic with continual use. Do not use if you have liver damage and check for contraindication with any pharmaceutical medications. Work with a qualified herbalist when using larger dosages. Boneset is not considered edible.

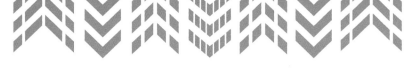

WILD GINGER

Asarum canadense
Asarum caudatum

I first meet wild ginger at the University of British Columbia with my herb class back in 2005. Growing below the damp, dappled shade canopy, she is a low-creeping rhizomatic mover. She has heart-shaped evergreen leaves and bell-shaped purple-brown flowers with three petals that bloom in April, growing into egg-shaped fruits. You can experience her lemon-ginger aroma when you crush the leaf.

Some websites say she is not edible and not recommended for consumption. This is always the challenge when you have conflicting information, although both species of wild ginger, *Asarum canadense* and *A. caudatum*, were administered as medicines by many Nations and Tribes. The roots were dried, ground, boiled until tender. Simmer for 20 to 30 minutes to make a syrup for coughs, stomach problems, indigestion, earaches, and colic. The leaf is antifungal and antibacterial and can be applied to cuts and sprains. A strong decoction was used as a contraceptive. Her leaf is diaphoretic for fevers and is helpful for gas and cramping during menses. She was also used as an herbal wash to cleanse the skin for rashes, chicken pox, and acne. The Algonquin of Quebec offered infused roots for convulsing infants. It is not completely clear if ginger root is antitumor or carcinogenic. Could the poison be in the dose?

 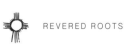

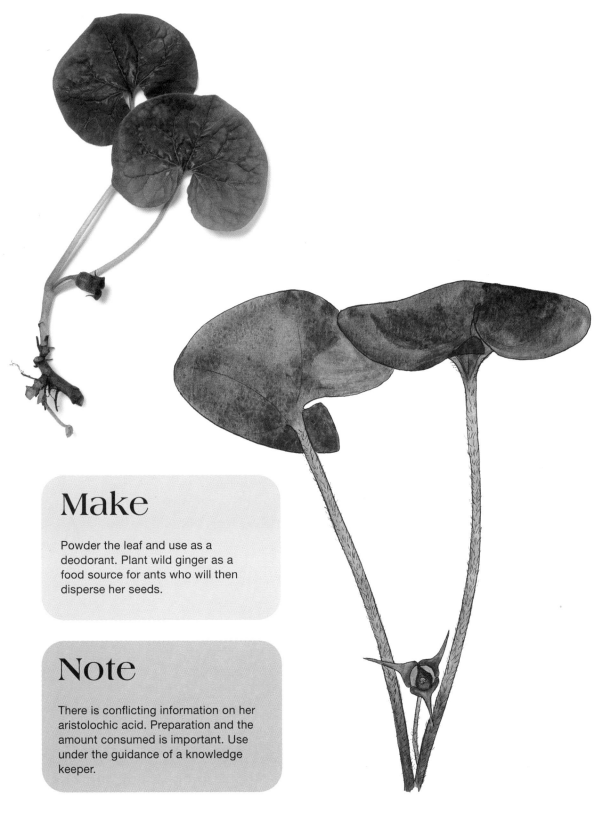

Make

Powder the leaf and use as a deodorant. Plant wild ginger as a food source for ants who will then disperse her seeds.

Note

There is conflicting information on her aristolochic acid. Preparation and the amount consumed is important. Use under the guidance of a knowledge keeper.

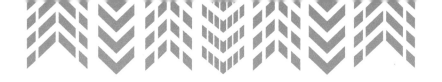

PARTRIDGEBERRY

Mitchella repens

I personally have never met partridgeberry and as I became curious about her gifts, I recognized again that our More-Than-Human-Kin offer so many teachings. She is a native plant that our Indigenous Nations have been walking with for centuries. It is a gift and privilege that our More-Than-Human-Kin share their medicine, their ability to bring relief, comfort, and healing. The most prevalent application was for women, supporting their menstruation cycles and for birthing. The Cherokee took partridgeberry monthly for menstrual pain and administered it to their cats and kittens. The Lenape People made infusions to strengthen the female reproductive organs. The Haudenosaunee ate the berries to prevent severe labor pains and to facilitate delivery, and they also made love medicine. The Ojibwe smoked the leaves during ceremonies.

Partridgeberry is listed on the United Plant Savers site as one of our native plants "to watch." As our native medicinal plants become more "popular," more stress is applied for commerce. Easy to grow, she adapts to both northern ranges and subtropical areas. She is found in Zones 3 to 9 in moist soil and full to part shade. Partridgeberry grows well from cuttings once established or from seed that has been planted in the summer for an overwinter, cold, moist stratification. Since her seed is hydrophilic, it cannot be stored and it may take until the second spring before she germinates. Related to the Rubiaceae, or coffee family, she is a creeping, shade-preferring, evergreen vine that makes a great ground cover. Her two little white flowers are fused to one calyx (ovary), and once both are pollinated creates one berry. Look for partridgeberry under pine forests, with her two little indents (scars) to properly identify the fruit.

When collecting, take only a little root, stem, leaves, and either some flower or berry, if available, to make fresh tea or a tincture. The red berry is edible, like a slightly sweet, astringent cucumber.

Partridgeberry is known as an emmenagogue, a diuretic, a parturient, and a styptic. She is also used for leg cramps, back pain, and to calm the nerves. She has been helpful for women who have experienced multiple miscarriages, and she is a tonic for infertility and menstrual cramps, urinary tract disorders, incontinence in children, digestive challenges like diarrhea, and painful urination. She has been used as a uterine tonic for heavy periods and after childbirth, miscarriage, or surgical abortion.

Make

For the last 4 to 6 weeks of pregnancy, make a tea with 1 tablespoon herb per 1 cup (240 ml) water. For tinctures, take 20 to 30 drops per day.

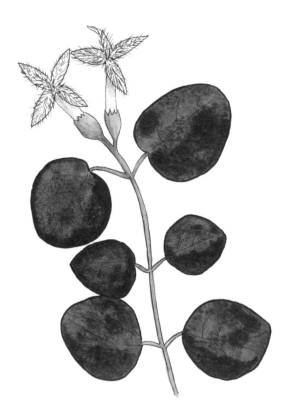

There are various herbs that are helpful for supporting the birth of our children. Partridgeberry tones the uterus and the nervous system as the birth approaches and is known as one of the safer partus-preparators herbs (herbs that help prepare for labor). Various resources have contradictory information regarding the first and second trimester; therefore, I highly recommend you reach out to an herbalist who can guide you through your decision on the most amazing journey we women experience.

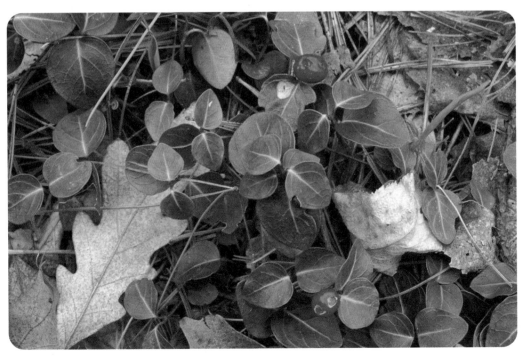

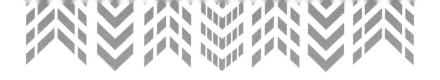

BLACK-EYED SUSAN

Rudbeckia hirta

Native to the east side of Turtle Island, black-eyed Susan surrounds my mother-in-law's garden, reminding me that the medicine we need is usually growing outside your door. In the National Library of Medicine an article on *Rudbeckia hirta* reported on a phytochemical investigation of her flower. A 5-lipoxygenase (5-LOX) inhibitor, she activates the immune response and contains antioxidants, supporting evidence of the ethnopharmacological use of her gifts in inflammatory conditions.

The first European settlers incorporated her medicine into their own herbal traditions from the generosity of the First Peoples' traditional medicines. The root is collected in the autumn and used to expel worms or assist for colds and stomach ailments. Black-eyed Susan is antimicrobial and diuretic. The root is more effective than echinacea in activating the immune system. She is an external wash for sores and snakebites. Be aware that the seeds are poisonous and some folks report sensitivity to her medicine.

Her daisy-like yellow flower typically reaches heights of 2 to 3 feet (61 to 91 cm). She is very adaptable and flourishes in diverse soil conditions. Black-eyed Susan is hardy and versatile, found in meadows, prairies, roadsides, and open woodlands from Canada to Mexico.

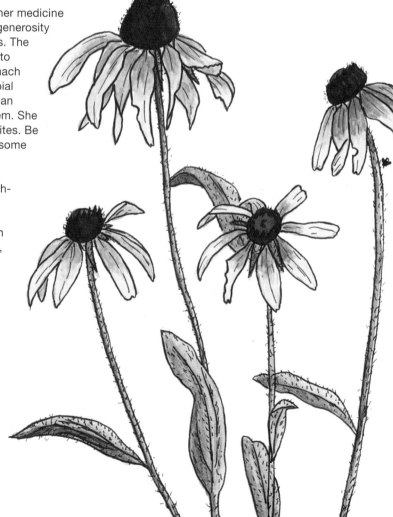

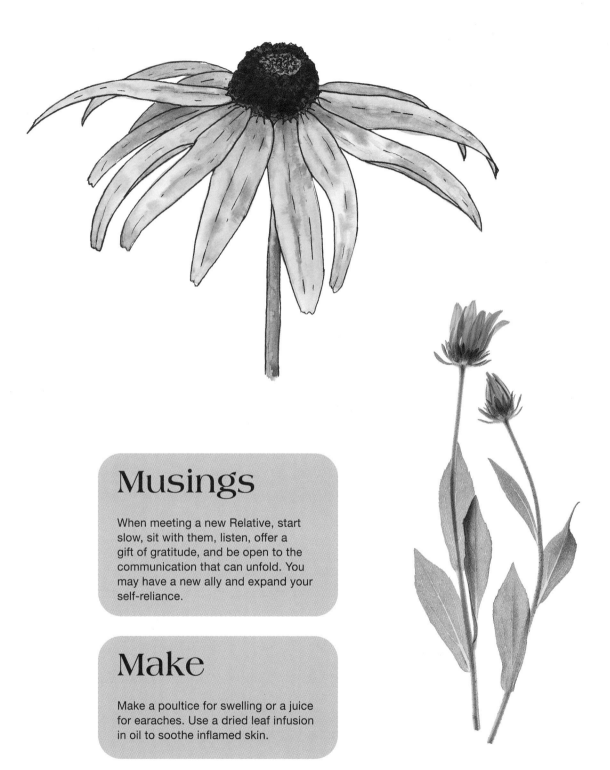

Musings

When meeting a new Relative, start slow, sit with them, listen, offer a gift of gratitude, and be open to the communication that can unfold. You may have a new ally and expand your self-reliance.

Make

Make a poultice for swelling or a juice for earaches. Use a dried leaf infusion in oil to soothe inflamed skin.

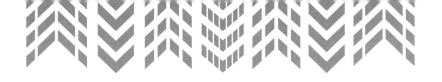

WAPATO

Sagittaria latifolia

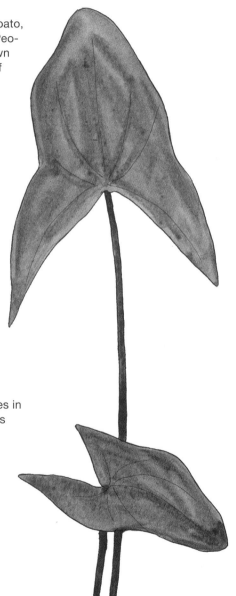

An aquatic herbaceous perennial, our More-Than-Human-Kin, wapato, with her arrowhead-shaped leaves, was observed by the Ojibwe People as a favorite food of ducks and geese. The edible corms, known as a *turion*, around the size of a walnut, are part of the structure of the rhizome that store energy for growth. Grown throughout Turtle Island down into Mexico, she is a valued food that can be boiled, dried, or mixed with maple sugar as candy. There is evidence from explorers' recorded accounts that families would own large patches of wapato. The corms, harvested in the autumn, would be exchanged for trade, as a currency for gambling, or stored for the winter months. The corms can be fire roasted, made into soup, or pounded into cakes. Other parts are edible, including the unfurled leaves and the stalks, which can be cooked like other greens. Before the flower blooms the immature rhizomes can be eaten raw or cooked. The edible white flower is delightful eaten raw for her minty flavor. Various parts of wapato were used for medicine and as a love charm.

It is great exercise for our toes to unearth the corms as we wade in marshy areas, swampy grounds, along lakeshores and the edges of streams and ditches. Wapato gathers nutrients as well as metals, so make sure the water is clean as you collect wapato's bluish, creamy white, or pinkish tubers. They are too bitter to eat raw, so peel the skin and cook to experience her starchy potato and corn-like flavor of roasted chestnuts.

Classified in the water plantain family (Alismataceae), wapato varies in size and shape. Thirty species of *Sagittaria* are an edible, nutritious carbohydrate, containing proteins, insoluble fiber, and various vitamins; she also contains diterpene glycoside, which may seriously upset your stomach. Prepare properly.

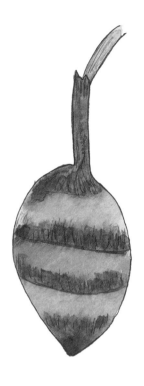

Look-alikes

Wapato's leaf, which has a distinct pointed V shape and is dark green with the veins running parallel, is similar to Italian arum (*Arum italicum*) and calla lily (*Zantedeschia aethiopica*).

Musings

Let's restore some of the traditional wetlands and bring back our native Rooted Nations to create habitat and food for our relatives, the muskrat and beaver.

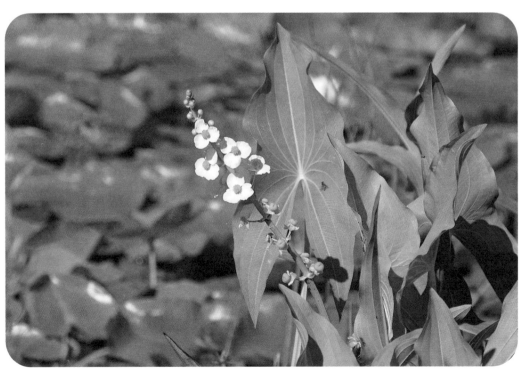

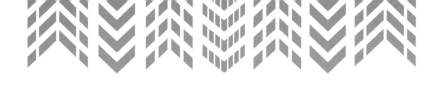

STAGHORN SUMAC

Rhus typhina
Rhus glabra

I love the adventure when I discover a plant that I have not met before. The key to foster and nurture a new relationship is to make sure you have clearly identified your new ally. There are eleven species of sumac the First Peoples forged a kinship with. We can see the complexity of Indigenous knowledge with the blending of other herbs as medicine. *Rhus typhina* was infused with chokecherry, oak, yellow birch, and dogwood for rheumatism by the Algonquin People of Quebec. The Diegueno, Kumeyaay, Ipai, Tipai, and Yuman People of the desert placed wads of *Rhus integrifolia* leaves in their mouth to alleviate thirst for long journeys on foot. The Cahuilla, also known as ʔívilʸuqaletem or Ivilyuqa-letem, infused leaves of *Rhus ovata* for coughs and chest pain. They dried the sumac berries and ground them into flour, and the fruit sap was used for sweetening. The Natchez made a poultice with the roots of *Rhus aromatica* for boils. The Coushatta who speak their native language Koasati, made decoctions of *Rhus copallinum* leaves for orthopedic and pediatric aid. The Keres Tribes infused the leaves of skunkbush sumac, *Rhus trilobata*, as an emetic and a stomach wash and infused the berries for a mouthwash.

Sumac has a long history as a food, medicine, implements for basketry, fiber, sunhats, mordant, tobacco mixes, pollen, bows, spear shafts, dyes, and ceremonial items. In Michael Moore's book, *Medicinal Plants of the Pacific West*, he suggests leaf powders for topical application as a gentle astringent for inflammations, herpes sores, wounds, and diaper rash. A cold infusion is best to extract the flavor without the tannins. Sumac's leaf and bark have been used for centuries for their tannins in the leather industry.

Rhus coriaria from the Mediterranean region is known as a spice, condiment, and flavoring agent along with a tradition medicine of the Middle East. Sumac fruits have been used in folk medicine for liver disease and the urinary system, to stimulate perspiration, and to reduce cholesterol. She can be applied externally for hemorrhoids, diarrhea, ulcers, eye inflammation, and wound healing. She contains a host of phytochemicals: flavonoids, tannins, polyphenolic compounds, and organic acids. Sumac is a powerful antioxidant, offering therapeutic benefits for cardiovascular disease, diabetes, and some cancers.

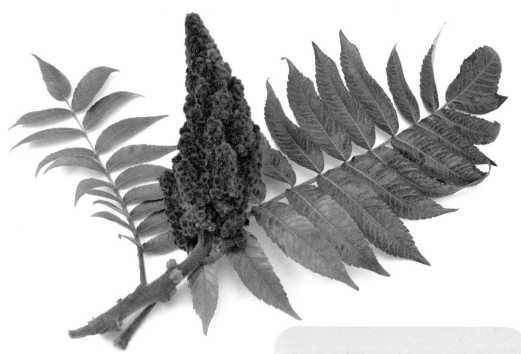

Sumac is known as a pioneer shrub, moving into disturbed sites and establishing herself in the landscape. Some species has velvety hairs on the branches but not on the bark. Her leaf is pinnately divided with a toothed edge and her leaves turn a bright red in the autumn. Her clusters of berries can be harvested into the winter months. New shoots can be eaten in the early spring; snap off and peel the outer skin to eat raw. Do not wash the berry clusters as you will lose the acidic, tart taste. Before collecting, identify which is the most flavorful fruit by licking your finger, placing it inside the vibrant red clusters, and tasting.

Make

Make a sun infusion and add various fresh fruits for a refreshing "lemonade." Dry the fruits and powder them to add to salads or minced meat to add in a lemony flavor.

Look-alikes

Watch out for look-alike poison sumac, *Toxicodendron vernix*. Poison sumac, like staghorn sumac, is in the cashew family, Anacardiaceae, which members grow clusters of white, yellow, or green flowers ripening to light green berries that hang down. Notice the cluster of poison sumac leaflets have smooth edges, which release an oily, intensely irritating toxin called urushiol. Urushiol is also found in poison ivy and poison oak. Wash immediately with soap and water. If the rash persists after a few days, contact medical assistance.

Note

Sumac contains latex. Do not use if you have allergies.

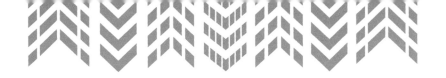

SUNCHOKE

Helianthus tuberosus

We find many species of *Helianthus* classified in the Asteraceae family. *Helianthus tuberosus* is one of the native tubers cultivated by our Indigenous Nations from the central and eastern parts of Turtle Island. The Apache made a poultice for a snake remedy by crushing the whole plant. The Hopi used her as spider bite medicine and as fodder for summer birds. The Meskwaki poulticed the flower blossoms for burns and the Keres Nation juiced the stem to apply to bleeding wounds. There is a thorough list in Moerman's ethnobotany book on the many applications of sunchoke, including as an anthelmintic, disinfectant, and antirheumatic and to treat pulmonary, dermatological treatment, pediatric, gynecological, cardiac, and gastrointestinal aid issues.

Many Nations honored this food by inviting sunchoke to participate in their ceremonies. They painted their faces with the oil from the seeds. They powdered the seeds and mixed them into cakes to combat fatigue while on a war party. The pith was used to light tobacco for their ceremonies or the stems used to make prayer sticks. In ceremonies, the blooms were used to honor our human existence on Earth. The number of flowers growing was a sign that there would be ample rain and a bountiful, generous harvest to celebrate another season on Mother Earth, a beautiful practice of reverence through observation.

Harvest her after the first frost. Some species do not store well, so harvest as needed for food. Sunchokes are yellow, crisp, and sweeter than potatoes because they contain a complex sugar know as inulin. This sugar breaks down more slowly during digestion and is considered good for diabetics requiring a low-starch diet.

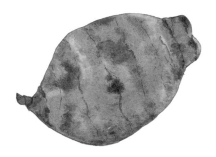

Make

Grate raw sunchokes to add to salads, make a creamy sunchoke soup, or steam with other vegetables. Sunchokes do not need to be peeled, simply scrub the outer skin well.

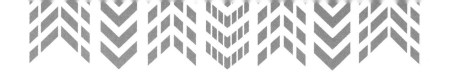

GINSENG

Panax quinquefolius

When driving north up through the canyons of the Fraser and Thompson Rivers area, I would see large dark tarp canopies covering the landscape: ginseng farms. With the overharvesting of ginseng in her natural landscape, we unfortunately interfered with the delicate balance of the evolution of our other relatives. In my experience, our More-Than-Human-Kin show us the importance of restoring our own equilibrium, and her gifts of healing and health were not meant to be over-consumed. Western science shows that the quality of ginseng differs greatly between a commercially grown ginseng and a wild ginseng. Are you able to find seeds and reintroduce them into our wild landscapes and reconcile with ginseng, the lands, and the waters?

Ginseng helps calm our anxiety when we have a nervous stomach from stress. She is an adaptogen, regulating our moods, an energy booster, antiviral, aphrodisiac, adrenal hormone stimulant, and supports the immune system. It is recommended to take ginseng only for one week to one month, then take a break. Search for local herbal support, and diversify applications and medicines to assist with any of the challenges you might be experiencing. I find "radical rest" sometime is the best medicine to rejuvenate our bodies.

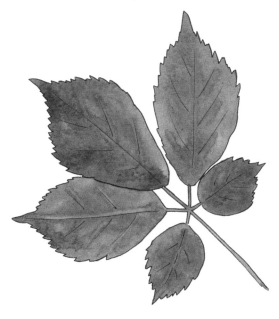

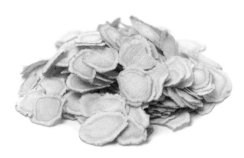

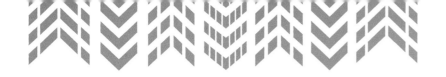

PRICKLY ASH

Zanthoxylum americanum

Prickly ash is known as the toothache plant. The Alabama Nations packed the inner bark around teeth with cavities. They were also known to use the bark for itchy skin, while the Comanche pulverized and powdered it for burns. The Lenape used the inner bark for heart medicine and the Haudenosaunee made a decoction to promote miscarriage, alleviate cramping, or expels worms. The Mohegan drank prickly ash bark tea three days on and then three days off, in small dosages. The Potawatomi used the root bark for gonorrhea and the Omaha prepared the fruits as a perfume for young men or made incense. The Seminole used *Zanthoxylum fagara* for bows and arrows.

Many other uses for *Zanthoxylum americanum* are listed by Indigenous Nations and Tribes for itchy skin, colds, pulmonary aid, sore throats, burns, fevers, back pain, kidney troubles, and rheumatism. *Z. clava-herculis* root was grated and used by the Houma Tribe for toothaches. *Zanthoxylum hirsutum* is known as "tingle tongue" because the leaf will eventually numb your tongue. The medicine moves stagnant conditions as she is a peripheral vasodilator.

Cardinal birds reseed the red berries from this small aromatic shrub, usually growing close to juniper. The fruits are collected for their spicy peppercorn citrus flavor; remove the black seed and dry for Szechuan cooking. You can harvest the husk, which has a slightly less intense flavor, without having to remove the seeds. This spice is heating, slightly numbing, and zingy. It's great for lamb or duck. Unripened seeds can be pickled and very young leaves can be eaten fresh. Start with small amounts of either tea or tincture made fresh or with dried bark.

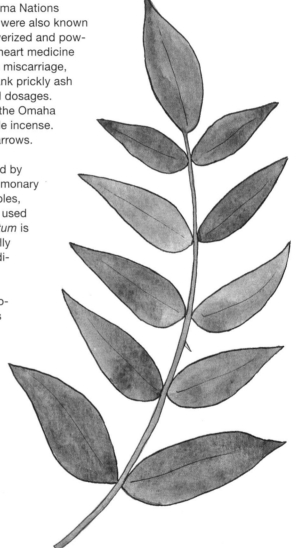

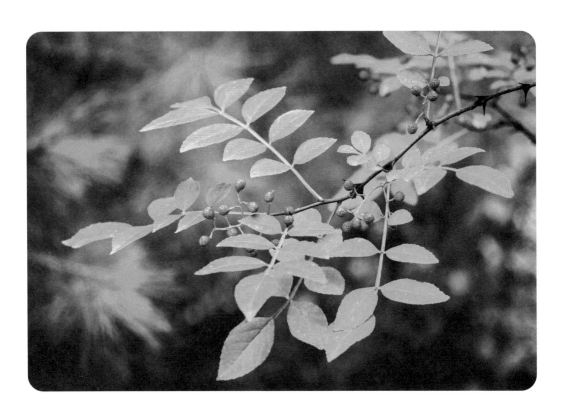

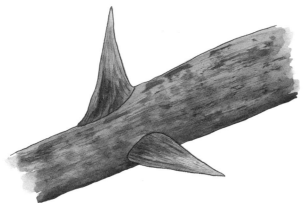

Note

Prickly ash bark is not recommended for folks on anticoagulant therapy. This medicine may irritate sensitive stomachs.

Make

Make a salt and pepper seasoning by heating equal parts salt and prickly ash husks/seeds for a few minutes until the salt turns brown. Remove from the heat and grind. For a cold formula, blend with yarrow and elderflower.

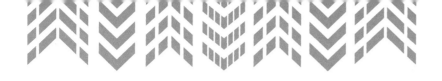

SLIPPERY ELM

Ulmus rubra

Growing upwards of 80 feet (24 m) with a wide canopy to shade our homes, slippery elm trees are our natural air conditioners. The Dakota, Omaha, Pawnee, and Ponca made mortar and pestle implements with the wood of *Ulmus americana* for grinding medicine and perfumes. The wood and fibers were used for cordage, baskets, and posts for their earth lodges. The inner bark was cooked with buffalo fat and prized as a special treat by children. Her seeds and buds are eaten by a variety of birds and wildlife.

Slippery elm medicine stimulates the mucous membrane linings and is helpful for various gynecological, dermatological, and gastrointestinal applications. I make a porridge with slippery elm when my digestive system is inflamed. She is a soothing, nutritive food when convalescing. Her demulcent properties have been helpful with folks who are experiencing colitis, gastritis, vaginitis, burns, varicose ulcers, hemorrhoids, dysentery, sensitive digestion, or diarrhea. Slippery elm is an excellent lubricant with her mucilaginous properties, relieving irritation and quieting our nervous system. She is a prebiotic that feeds the good bacteria in our guts and reduces the growth of pathogens.

Collecting the inner bark is a delicate process to prevent damage and spreading of diseases like Dutch elm. It is best left to professional wildcrafters who pass on generational knowledge and use this to economically support their families and communities. Collecting the bark can be done any time of year, although spring is best when the sap is moving nutrients, sugars, and mucilage. Leave harvested trees for a few years so she has time to repair. Reach out to your local Indigenous community to honor this ancient medicine that gives freely when properly respected.

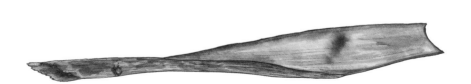

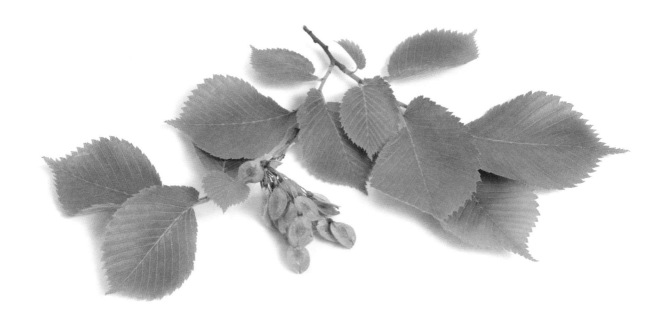

Make

Form a paste by mixing the powder with enough boiling water for a poultice for external use on boils, abscesses, and ulcers. Make a tea or porridge by mixing hot water with 1 to 4 teaspoons (5 to 20 g) powdered inner bark and eat three times a day. You can purchase capsules or make your own. Consider blending it with peppermint, licorice root, marshmallow root, or aloe vera extract. A combination increases her beneficial gifts. Make a tea for her gelatinous structure, which calms sore throats and coughs, adding honey to sweeten.

Note

Slippery elm slows the absorption of supplements and medications. Leave 2 hours between consumption.

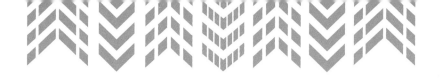

HAZELNUT

Corylus americana
Corylus cornuta
Corylus cornuta var. *californica*

Bagaan (Ojibwe for nut, hazelnut, or peanut) are a nut I live for! Many Nations had a relationship with hazelnut as medicine, gathering it for winter stores and for trade. My ancestors ate hazelnut during their seasonal cycle and it is comforting to be reminded of this connection with cultural foods. Eaten raw, hazelnuts move the bowels, slow weight gain, lower cholesterol, balance insulin, heal the heart, lower inflammation, and increase sperm count. The Haudenosaunee People crushed the nutmeat and mixed it with cornmeal and beans or berries to make bread. The Chippewa and Ojibwe made black dyes when boiled with butternut (*Juglans cinerea*).

One of her superpowers is manganese superoxide dismutase, an antioxidant enzyme that decreases oxidative stress and may reduce the risk of cancer. Her many life-giving nutrients, including vitamin E, polyphenol compounds, unsaturated fatty acids, and fiber, contribute to increasing diversity of microbes in the digestive tract, helping with bowel movements. Most of the antioxidants in hazelnuts are found in the skin. The fatty oleic acid has beneficial effects on insulin sensitivity.

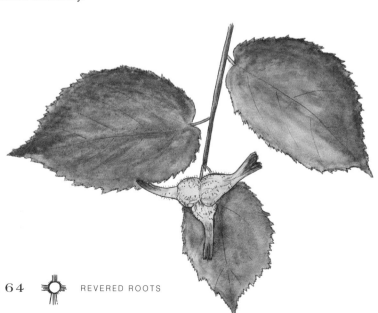

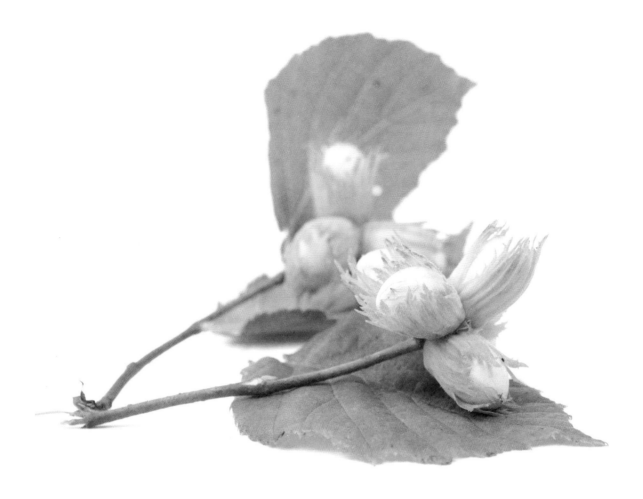

Note

If you have allergies to mugwort pollen, peanuts, Brazil nuts, birch pollen, or macadamia nuts, you may have allergies to hazelnut.

Make

Make a tasty treat by coating hazelnuts with chocolate, or sprinkle on spices like cinnamon or cayenne for either a sweet or spicy snack.

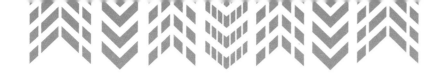

COREOPSIS

Coreopsis bigelovii

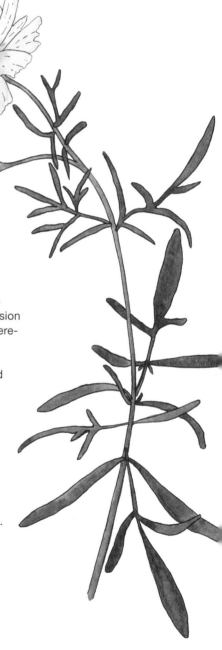

On my father's side of my lineage, there were two cousins with the same first name. It was confusing, so one cousin took the *e* out of Bigelow. I was stunned to find *Coreopsis bigelovii* listed in Moerman's ethnobotany book. The species epithet *bigelovii* is named in honor of Dr. John Milton Bigelow, an American physician and botanist (1804–1878.) I appreciate fresh-cut flowers, and coreopsis is a gorgeous native prairie plant that offers cheery, daisy-like blooms all summer long, thriving through sweltering heat and direct sunlight. Colors range from gold, yellow, and orange and there are many cultivars to choose from. It is known to make great dye colors.

Coreopsis is native to both Turtle Island and the southern continent known as *Abya Yala*, named by the Indigenous People of Panama and Columbia. The Kuna speak of their home as "the living land that flourishes." The Nuna People of the Tehachapi Valley, in California, chewed coreopsis stems for her sweet juice or cooked the whole plant in grease and salt. The Cherokee created red coloring or made an infusion with the root for diarrhea. The Navajo and Ramah honored coreopsis as a ceremonial medicine plant.

The root of *Coreopsis tinctoria*, a similar species, was taken as a panacea and as a "life medicine" by the Navajo People. The Zuni infused the whole plant except the root for women desiring a female baby. The National Library of Medicine reports that *C. tinctoria* was used to treat diarrhea, internal pain, and bleeding. Other applications include for liver diseases and diabetes. You can make a flower infusion for hypertension. The pharmacological studies indicate she has antioxidant and antidiabetic properties, among other benefits. She is rich in flavonoids to support good health.

Coreopsis grows in full sun for 6 to 8 hours a day; some varieties are drought and soil tolerant with little maintenance. Her leaf's aroma reminds me of anise. Her blooms attract birds, bees, and butterflies. Deadhead or cut regularly for continuous bloom from early summer into fall. Add a little compost each

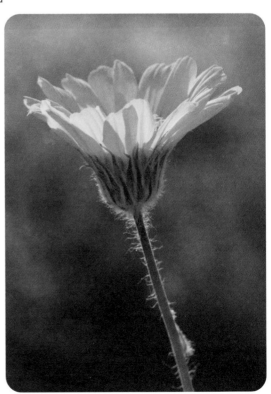

spring, grow for three to five years, then divide and replant into new areas or reseed. Save her seeds in paper bags and store in a cool, dry place. It's best to seed in the fall to support stratification or place in the fridge to stimulate.

Coreopsis bigelovii has yellow blooms and prefers open woodland, grassland, and the desert, blooming in June. There are dozens of species of coreopsis, so check for a native that grows in your ecosystem. I love the *C. grandiflora* cultivar 'Double the Sun', with her orange-yellow blooms. It reminds me of the orange color that symbolizes the lost children who never returned from residential schools.

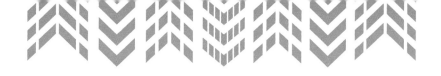

GINKGO

Ginkgo biloba

Driving through one of our city neighborhoods I saw the most stunning bright, vibrant yellow tree expressing her glory in the fading season. I was amazed to find a *Ginkgo biloba* tree and the possibility of collecting her leaf for medicine. I marked down the address and the following summer before the leaves turned yellow, I knocked on the owner's door to ask permission, which, thankfully, I was granted. The ginkgo tree is only a living representative of a group of gymnosperms, a living fossil dating back to the time of the Jurassic period. In the early autumn before her leaf changes color, we can gather her green leaf medicine and food from the fruit nut.

Thanks to the notes from my teacher, Don Ollsin, I learned that the molecules of ginkgo are so small they have the ability to pass through our capillaries. This explains her ability to be so helpful for the brain, heart, legs, eyes, and ears. As we age, blood flow decreases to the brain. European studies show that ginkgo is a circulatory stimulant, energy enhancer, and increases blood flow. She has been said to prevent blood clots from forming in the arteries, prevents and treats strokes, and improves memory and mental prowess. Ginkgo is effective in treating tinnitus and vertigo and has been administered for asthma for thousands of years in China.

Ginkgo is a wonderful ally for us as we age. Claudication, when cholesterol builds up in the arteries in calf muscles, can cause lameness, pain, cramping, and weakness in the elderly. To treat, try 40 mg of ginkgo three times a day, as it may give great relief over standard treatments. Cerebral insufficiency describes a collection of symptoms experienced in our elderly folk. Ginkgo may be the medicine needed for difficulties of concentration, absent-mindedness, confusion, lack of energy, tiredness, depressive mood, dizziness, and headaches.

As we age, blood flow also decreases to the eyes, in particular the retina, and if starved of blood it deteriorates, causing macular degeneration. The suggested dosage is 80 mg taken twice a day to improve vision. For age-related cochlear deafness, take 80 mg twice a day.

Collect the fruit in the fall, after the first frost. It contains a nut that is eaten in a porridge and is considered a delicacy to be served at a feast. Be mindful extracting the fruit, as it is very irritating to the skin. It was traditionally placed in water (or buried) and fermented for a few weeks to decompose. Once you extract the nut, roast or boil it for tea. It is a restorative food for ear health, bladder irritation, coughs, excessive mucus, intestinal worms, and gonorrhea and can be made into a poultice for infections. The nuts must be cooked as they are considered toxic if consumed raw.

 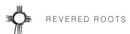

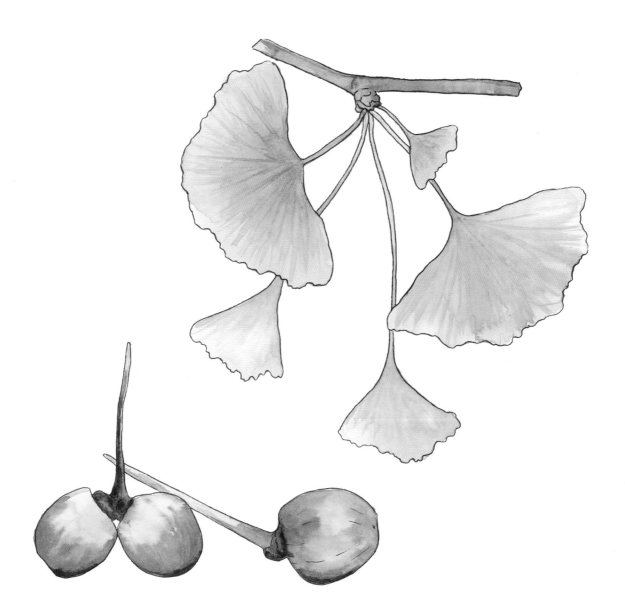

Make

To serve the nuts, cook 1 cup (165 g) rice and 10 to 15 nuts in 2½ cups (600 ml) water. Slowly heat until tender. Then, remove the nuts and serve with honey, butter, or olive oil.

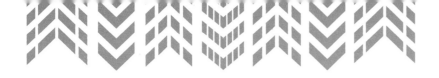

HONEY AND PROPOLIS

The time to check your hives for fully ripened honey is July to mid-September. Our little winged kin will cap the honey cells with a layer of wax to let you know. When you find the majority of cells are capped, this is your opportunity to harvest. Honey is a complex assortment of enzymes, trace minerals, organic acids, antibiotic agents, and hormones. She is also filled with vitamins A, B, C, D, E, and K. In particular, vitamin D and the sugars in honey help with the absorption of calcium. Honey is helpful for kidney and liver disorders, stimulates circulation, and eases cold symptoms. A spoonful of local honey taken daily is reported to help build immunity to seasonal allergies.

Yet another gift from the hive is propolis, of which we say, "cleans, seals, and heals" wounds. Propolis is created by the bees that have collected resin from leaf buds and flowers. The composition varies according to plant species, geography, climate, when collected, and the species of honeybees and flora. Propolis from bees here on Turtle Island, or around the world in Egypt, Cuba, Brazil, and Russia, will contain different compounds that align with the local ecosystem to help keep the honeybees healthy. The resin is processed by the enzymes from the bee's glands, which make a "bee glue" to protect and seal the hive from microbes and other invaders. Broad clinical applications of propolis show antioxidant, anti-inflammatory, antimicrobial, analgesic, antidepressant, immunomodulation, and even anticancer properties.

We Two-Leggeds have been using bee propolis medicinally, internally, and externally for centuries. The ancient Egyptians, Greeks, and Romans used her for wound healing, mouth ulcers, and throat infections. Today, we have extended her applications to skin care, dental health, digestion, and immune support. She is effective in promoting the regeneration of collagen, cartilage, bone, and dental pulp.

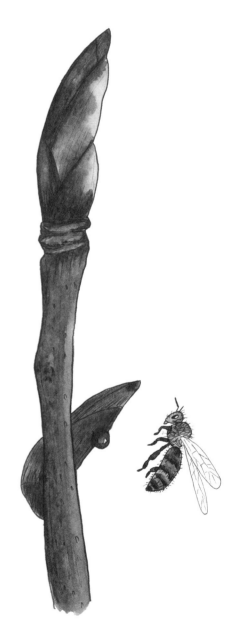

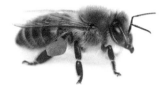

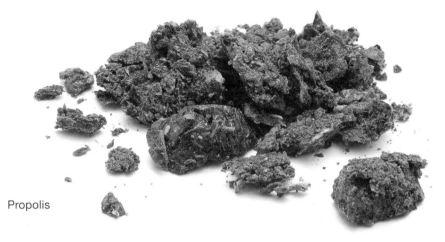

Propolis

Nutrients like flavonoids contribute to propolis's antibacterial, antiviral, antifungal, and anti-inflammatory properties. Propolis stimulates the macrophages, the immune cells responsible for the defense against microbial pathogens, to develop antibodies. This disrupts the proliferation of bacteria by inhibiting cell division and by destroying the bacteria's cell structure while reducing the life and spread of pathogens internally and externally. The research is fascinating, revealing how our environment produces the medicines that we need locally. Get to know your local beekeeper.

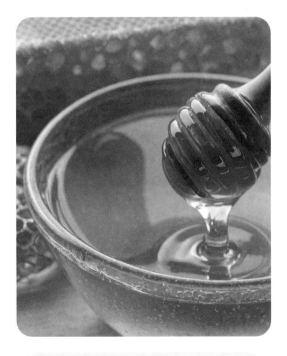

Bee pollen is another gift from honey-bees that can be used as a replacement for protein supplements.

Make

Make a propolis tincture with 190 proof alcohol.

MILKWEED

Asclepias tuberosa
Asclepias asperula
Asclepias speciosa

My dear mother-in-law would adopt monarch butterfly (*Danaus plexippus*) eggs and bring them in the house so our winged friends could not eat the eggs. Once they hatched and were growing as a caterpillar, she would feed them fresh milkweed leaves until they formed a chrysalis. I was blessed to witness a monarch butterfly come out of its cocoon. Last year I saw fewer than ten butterflies. Milkweed is the key species for their survival and their only host plant. Without milkweed, there are no more monarch butterflies.

Asclepias was named to honor Asklepios, the Greek god of medicine. Both our Indigenous Nations and early physicians valued *Asclepias tuberosa*'s root for pleurisy and other ailments. This species does not contain the latex juice we find in other species. She prefers full sun and sandy soil for the best medicines. Collect the root the first week of October to dry for teas, or tincture fresh root in 40 percent alcohol. Her gift is to equalize the circulation and is useful for bronchitis; catarrh; diarrhea; and harsh, rough, or sensitive skin. Milkweed is helpful medicine for chronic rheumatism, eczema, and dysentery.

More than a hundred species of milkweed grow throughout Turtle Island and Southern Africa. Various Nations made medicine from the roots of *Asclepias speciosa*, showy milkweed. She was used for gastrointestinal complaints, pain, coughs, kidney ailments, and as a contraceptive. The taste of milkweed's inner latex ranges from mild to bitter depending on the species, serving as a protection against grazing animals. The milky latex was applied to warts and used as an antiseptic for healing sores, cuts, and ringworm. The latex was also dried and hardened to be chewed for gum. Milkweed seeds were consumed as a gentle laxative. The silky coma fluff attached to the seed was used as a fiber for clothing, ceremonial items, thread, stuffing for beds and pillows, belts, and infant diapers. A decoction of the seeds was used to pull out the venom from snakebites. She is also known as pleurisy root, and in large doses milkweed works as an emetic and a purgative. However, unless you are working with a trained herbalist, it is best to use her in small amounts. As an edible, properly cook the young milkweed sprouts by boiling. Taste a small amount to make sure you don't react. Collect the sprouts from

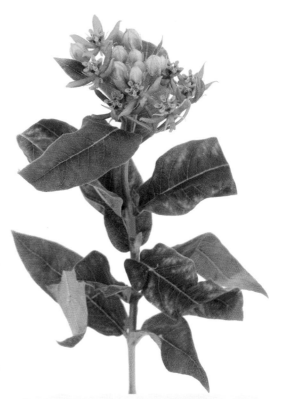

spring to fall, all the while remembering that we were an integral aspect of the ecosystems to support abundance life. Collect responsibly and help disperse the seeds.

You can directly sow milkweed seeds in the fall. The seedlings will emerge the following summer. Nectar from the flowers feeds many more diverse, winged species in addition to the monarch butterfly. Declining habitat due to widely separated nature spaces, suburban development, overgrazing livestock, fire suppression, pesticides and insecticides, and the introduction of nonnatives impact the survival of butterflies, our flying flowers. Abundant nectar is essential as it determines how many eggs will be laid. Butterflies are not just beautiful pollinators. All stages of the butterfly's life cycle provides food for birds, reptiles, and amphibians.

Look-alikes

Dogbane (*Apocynum* species) looks similar and is poisonous.

Note

Asclepias contains toxic resinoids and glycosides, and may overstimulate the heart. The latex may cause irritation to the skin.

Make

Steep a decoction of 1 teaspoon milkweed to 1 cup (240 ml) boiling water and take 2 to 3 ounces (56 to 84 ml) three times a day.

Make sure you grow your native species, not *Asclepias curassavica*, which is a native to the tropics and loved by monarch butterflies. Unfortunately, this species does not die back over winter in milder climates and hosts the protozoan parasite *Ophryocystis elektroscirrha*. The monarch ingests the parasite and when they hatch from their chrysalises, they are covered in spores, making them weaker and not able to fly south to Mexico or live long.

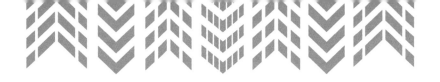

AMERICAN CHESTNUT

Castanea dentata

Eating local is relational, an act of belonging to place. We are nourished and informed by the land and water. When one of our relatives is threatened by introduced pathogens like the blight fungus *Cryphonectria parasitica*, it has a devastating effect on the web of life, including horse chestnut. One-fourth of all hardwoods used to be American chestnut. Now considered a functionally extinct species, American chestnut cannot reproduce without human intervention. The Cherokee Nation and the American Chestnut Foundation are collaborating and researching ways to breed with the blight-resistant Chinese chestnut (*Castanea mollissima*). The beloved American chestnut was a staple for the First Peoples, who shared with the settlers her plethora of gifts of medicine, dyes, wood, and commerce for the newcomers.

American chestnut, a member of the beech family, grows up to 115 feet (35 m) at full maturity. The trees are found mostly in sunny wooded areas and along edges and roadsides of the Appalachian range. In the month of June we can experience her canopy of odoriferous catkins providing an ocean of pollen for our winged relatives. The catkins give way to her bounty of sharp globes, curled up like a hedgehog protecting a delicious, edible nut. By collecting leaves and bark, teas were made for various ailments like typhoid and stomach pain. Aged leaves made tea for heart challenges and young sprouted leaves for old sores. The Haudenosaunee made insecticides, dermatological aids to wash an itch, and powdered wood for diaper rash. The Mohicans applied an infusion of leaves for colds, whooping cough, and rheumatism. The chestnut's oil was extracted and sometimes mixed with bear grease for a hair treatment. The bark was also administered to dogs who were experiencing worms. Made into flavoring for foods, beverages, bread, cakes, pies, puddings, soups and sauces, she is an important food source and medicine.

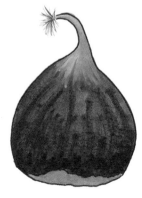

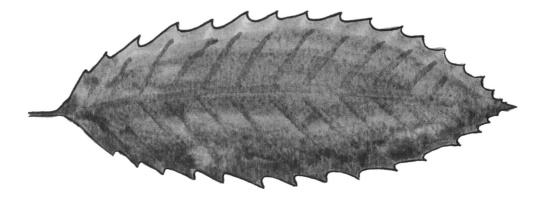

Musings

As the Europeans arrived and settled, we are reminded of their community gatherings to collect and process the chestnuts as our Indigenous neighbors have done for thousands of years. As we reclaim acts of service to our ecosystems, we can restore our local foods and move away from the industrial corporate food system that applies a plethora of pesticides, insecticides, and fungicides, and plants genetically modified seeds. Where will our migrating winged kin find their food?

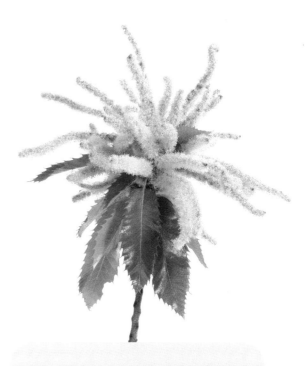

Make

Make a cough syrup with boiled chestnut leaves, mullein, and sweetener. The chestnuts can be used as a coffee substitute, ground for baking breads, or blended with corn.

With a plethora of gifts that supported lifeways for thousands of years, let's celebrate and eat some of our native nuts, such as butternut, hazelnut, groundnut, pecans, walnuts, pine nut, beech, and hickory, along with this beloved "cradle to casket" nut tree.

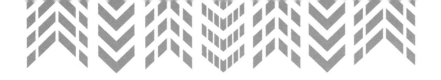

HYDRANGEA

Hydrangea arborescens

My herbology teacher, Don Ollsin, would say, "Whoever is growing around you might be your medicine." Perhaps you have some pretty hydrangeas in your garden? The Cherokee have a list of ailments that they dispensed hydrangea roots and rhizomes for. She was used as an abortifacient (causing abortion), antiemetic (preventing vomiting), burn treatment, cancer treatment for tumors, dermatological aid (diagnosis and treatment of skin disorders), gastrointestinal aid, purgative, disinfectant, hypotensive (decreasing blood pressure), liver aid, help for sore and swollen muscles, and a stimulant.

Hydrangea is Greek for "water vessel." Amazingly, there is a fossil record of her here on Turtle Island 70 million years ago. She is well known as an ornamental, but her roots and rhizomes are used as medicine to treat wounds, kidneys, the prostate gland, and the bladder. In Japan, *ama-cha* tea is made with *Hydrangea serrata* to honor the Buddha's birthday on April 8. In Korea, hydrangea tea is called *sugukcha*. In Nepal, hydrangea is decocted for colds and indigestion. When introduced to Europe, English folklore reported that growing hydrangea close to your house would make you unlucky in love.

Hydrangea root helps increase the absorption of calcium, reducing the formation of kidney stones and helping to remove them. She is helpful for autoimmune disorders and has a relative in China, *Dichroa febrifuga*, which has been used as a powerful antimalarial medicine because it contains the constituent febrifugine, which is considered a hundred times more potent than quinine.

A 2003 study published in *Bioscience, Biotechnology, and Biochemistry* reported that hydrangea root extract contains more antioxidants than milk thistle seeds and turmeric combined. The constituent halofuginone demonstrated the root's ability to interfere with autoimmune pathogens while at the same time not suppressing the immune system. Side effects with her use are uncommon. Like any diuretic, the medicine increases output of urine, flushes electrolytes, and lowers blood pressure. Do not use long term. Make sure you have the right species of hydrangea for medicine making—*Hydrangea arborescens*.

 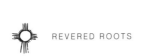

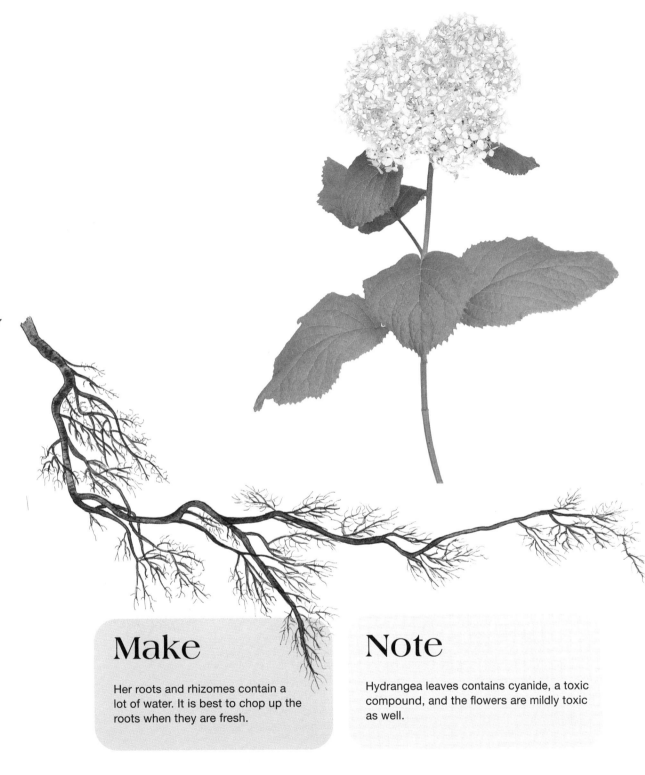

Make

Her roots and rhizomes contain a lot of water. It is best to chop up the roots when they are fresh.

Note

Hydrangea leaves contains cyanide, a toxic compound, and the flowers are mildly toxic as well.

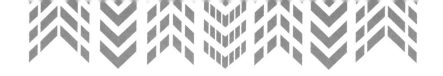

MARSHMALLOW

Althaea officinalis

All the flowers of the mallow family (Malvaceae) are beautiful and have many benefits. The genus *Malva* is derived from the Latin *mollis* or the Greek *malake*, meaning "soft," relating to her soothing and beneficial qualities. During the Middle Ages, she was grown in European monasteries. Marshmallow originally grew abundantly along the floodplains of the Nile. She grows alongside waterways like marshes, seas, and other damp areas and can reach a height of 2 to 4 feet (61 to 122 cm). Marshmallow is a decorative perennial with hairy kidney-shaped leaves and large pale pink, white, or purple blooms. Her long white taproot anchors her into Mother Earth to hold her upright.

Marshmallow therapeutics work on inflammation of the alimentary canal (the passage from mouth to anus) as well as for the kidney and bladder, ulceration of the stomach and duodenum, hiatus hernia, dry coughs, open wounds, cystitis, diarrhea, mucous membranes, boils, abscesses, and a buildup of mucus in the respiratory system or stomach.

Like a protective film on inflamed mucosa, marshmallow root is a soothing demulcent for irritated tissues, producing an immediate effect and faster regeneration. The root contains 25 to 35 percent mucilage, plus flavonoids, tannins, scopoletin (lowers high blood pressure), polysaccharides, asparagine, and pectin. Use her externally as an emollient to soften and soothe the skin. Marshmallow's gel-like consistency coats and protects inflamed nerve endings. She reduces or suppresses urinary stones and is an antitussive (relieves coughs), a diuretic, and an expectorant. Even though she has healing attributes for the many systems of the body, she has a specific relationship to the kidneys, due to her salty, mucilaginous properties. Both the flower and the leaves contain mucilage, flavonoids, and coumarin. The leaf also contains salicylic and phenolic acids.

Marshmallow root is best to dig up in the fall and winter to gather the highest content of mucilaginous properties. Collect leaves after flowering. You can eat all parts of the marshmallow. Like most members of the mallow family, hollyhock (*Alcea rosea*) and common mallow or cheeseweed (*Malva neglecta*) are also edible. The seeds, leaves, and flowers can be added to salads and the leaves steamed like kale. It was eaten by the Romans, the Egyptians, in Arabic-speaking countries, and in India. Marshmallow is an important herb in the Indian Ayurveda healing tradition. The root is offered to reduce Vata (dry constitutional type) and increase Kapha (wet constitutional type), as she is energetically cold, sweet-tasting, and moistening.

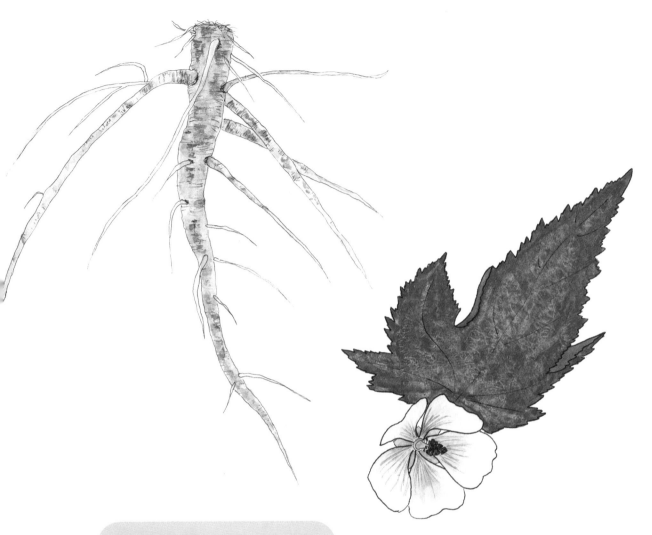

Make

Steep marshmallow tea blended with fennel, coriander, cumin, and orange peel. For sore throats, make a gargle solution with the leaf and flower or make a cold infusion of the root. Cook the root with honey and form into soft balls for children to suck on or create lozenges. The flowers make a great expectorant syrup for coughs.

Note

Drink at least 1 cup (240 ml) of liquids when ingesting. Marshmallow will slow the absorption of pharmaceuticals. It's best to take a prescription medication 1 hour prior to or several hours after consuming marshmallow.

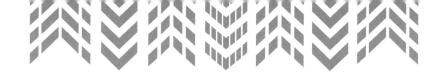

CRABAPPLE

Malus fusca

On a cold February day, I witnessed ice-covered, red crabapples drooping on her branches, and a woodpecker pounding on her frozen fruit. I am grateful for the person who planted her. I see very few of our Rooted Nations, such as the crabapple growing here in the city. Dr. Luschiim Arvid Charlie shares in his book *Luschiim's Plants* that grouse and pheasants' favorite place to roost is under a crabapple tree. She is a plant that offers life to many of our relatives: birds, bees, bears, deer, and other wildlife.

A very sour, tangy, tart, small apple, crabapples are delicious and a highly prized food for Coast Salish Peoples. *Malus fusca* is picked when green and stored in masterful, exquisite western red cedar bentwood boxes while immersed in water, ripening over time. The Nations would also eat them fresh with eulachon grease. The stored crabapples would be shared when feasting, celebrating, and hosting ceremony and were traded as well.

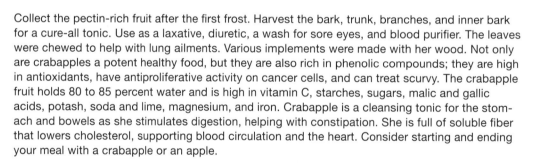

Collect the pectin-rich fruit after the first frost. Harvest the bark, trunk, branches, and inner bark for a cure-all tonic. Use as a laxative, diuretic, a wash for sore eyes, and blood purifier. The leaves were chewed to help with lung ailments. Various implements were made with her wood. Not only are crabapples a potent healthy food, but they are also rich in phenolic compounds; they are high in antioxidants, have antiproliferative activity on cancer cells, and can treat scurvy. The crabapple fruit holds 80 to 85 percent water and is high in vitamin C, starches, sugars, malic and gallic acids, potash, soda and lime, magnesium, and iron. Crabapple is a cleansing tonic for the stomach and bowels as she stimulates digestion, helping with constipation. She is full of soluble fiber that lowers cholesterol, supporting blood circulation and the heart. Consider starting and ending your meal with a crabapple or an apple.

Crabapple trees are found close to water, in moist woods, along the edges of streams and rivers, and in estuaries. Botanists believe Pacific crabapple traveled from across the Bering Land Bridge between Siberia and Alaska during the last ice age. It is believed apples originated in Kazakhstan, in Central Asia east of the Caspian Sea, arriving in Europe around the 1500s. In medieval times, herbalism was a blend of superstition and fact. Many created their own remedies, praying to the gods for blessings. If the remedy did not work, they concocted a new one with new incantations. An anonymous written remedy was the "Nine Herbs Charm," recorded in the *Lacnunga* manuscript from the eleventh century. Originating from Anglo-Saxon text, the manuscript, Harley 585, today resides in the British Museum. Let's replant the guild of nine herbs—mugwort, stinging nettle, plantain, lamb's crest, betony, chamomile, fennel, and chervil—around the crabapple tree. We'll say our prayers and make some good medicine.

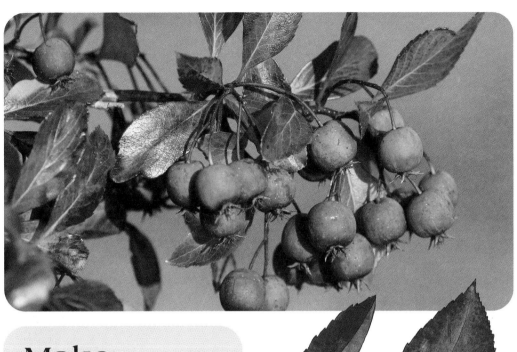

Make

Crabapples make lovely jellies, hard cider, vinegar, and butter.

Musings

Graft crabapples from a heritage species and grow a hedgerow fence.

Note

The bark contains cyanide, so use sparingly. It's best to avoid eating too many crabapples raw because it could cause stomach upset.

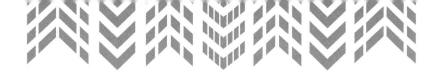

BLACK COHOSH

Actaea racemosa

Black bugbane, another name for black cohosh, is an herbal medicine of the Western Woodland Natives of Turtle Island. She has an affinity with the cerebrospinal and reproductive systems. We can see the influence and exchange of knowledge as the Indigenous People started to infuse black cohosh root in alcohol. The alcohol infusion was taken for rheumatism pain, colds, coughs, hives, constipation, and fatigue. The Cherokee used it to stimulate menstruation, as the root has strong abortifacient properties. The name *cohosh* is an Algonquin word connected to pregnancy and administered as a parturient (to bring forth) in the last stages of labor. She was also used to increase the flow of breast milk. The Lenape People made a tonic blended with elecampane (*Inula helenium*) and stone root (*Collinsonia canadensis*). The Haudenosaunee made a decoction of her root to apply externally in baths and steams for rheumatism. The Mi'kmaq and Penawapskewi used the root for the kidneys.

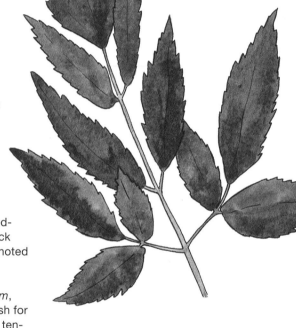

Actaea (formerly *Cimicifuga racemosa*) is a member of the buttercup family and was introduced as a homeopathic medicine back in 1856. It has similar medicine to *Pulsatilla*. Black cohosh, with her dark, matted, interwoven roots has been noted to help lift intense emotional states.

The herbalist Matthew Wood, in *The Book of Herbal Wisdom*, shares that his patients have had success with black cohosh for whiplash and fibromyalgia. Black cohosh helps release the tension that is bound up in the trapezius muscles. There are many documented cases of black cohosh efficacy, although Western science reports otherwise. The Cochrane Group did a meta-analysis of 152 studies on black cohosh and her effect on just vasomotor symptoms (hot flashes). They only assessed sixteen reports and stated in their conclusion that black cohosh did not help with hot flashes and it was "unclear [for] other routes of administration or types of preparation."

Consider growing these stunning flowering relatives for your home garden, sit with her, and ask for her assistance.

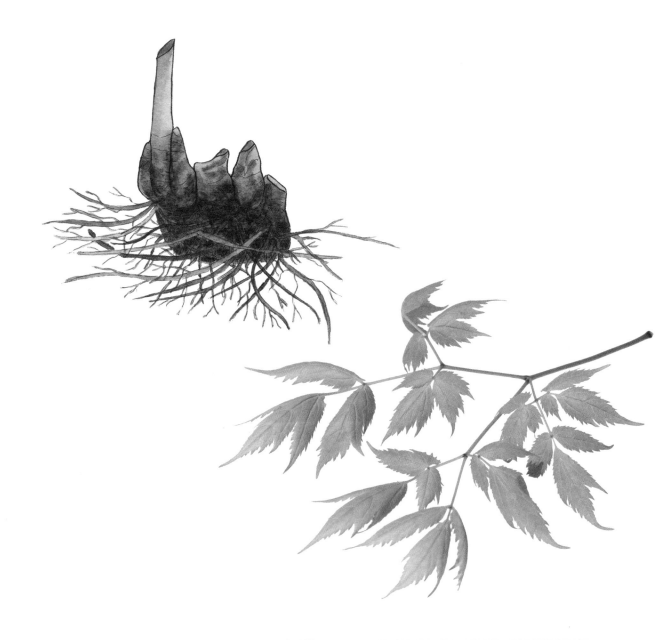

Make

Dig up the fresh root, chop, and
infuse in brandy or vodka. Infuse a
flower essence when in bloom around
the month of July.

Note

Very small drops are advised. Black cohosh
tea and capsules can be aggravating.
Consider using a homeopathic remedy
of black cohosh.

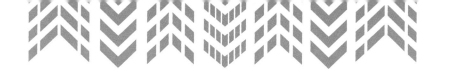

FENNEL

Foeniculum vulgare

Two decades ago, I wandered through a back alley to find a small forest of fennel growing. I remember feeling immense joy to see her growing wild and free, but the next time I went to visit, she was flattened by a large trucking container. Just like that, she was gone.

Fennel is an ancient cultural plant from the Mediterranean and was spread throughout Europe by the Romans. She is used in Traditional Chinese Medicine for longevity. We can see the exchange that occurred between the new settlers and Native Peoples as the Cherokee used fennel for children's flatulence, colic, colds, and as a tonic, and the Pomo Tribe made a tea for an eyewash or chewed the seeds for an upset stomach. I dispense fennel seeds any time my daughter has an upset stomach.

Fennel grows worldwide and is a very helpful herb for digestion, bloating, gas, heartburn, and colic. Fennel seeds are antispasmodic, calming the smooth muscles and activating peristalsis to keep everything moving in the digestive tract. Fennel contains coumarin, flavonoids like rutin, and sterols. She alleviates coughs and upper respiratory congestion. She is antimicrobial, aromatic, anticoagulant, and a rubefacient (causing cutaneous vasodilation in the treatment of pain for various musculoskeletal conditions). Fennel seeds support the kidneys and liver after childbirth and once the breast milk is flowing, new mothers can eat or drink fennel tea to support breast milk production.

Growing to 5 to 6 feet (1.5 to 1.8 m) tall, fennel is a perennial with feathery green leaves and hollow stems. A member of the carrot family, she has an umbel cluster of tiny yellow flowers that the bees and pollinators love. Collect the greenish gray seeds in early fall before they turn brown. Taste her warming, juicy, plump, pungent, sweet taste of licorice. Fennel has allelopathic tendencies and produces chemicals that adversely affect nearby plants, particularly the nightshade family, beans, basil, and cucumbers. Be mindful when planting in your garden.

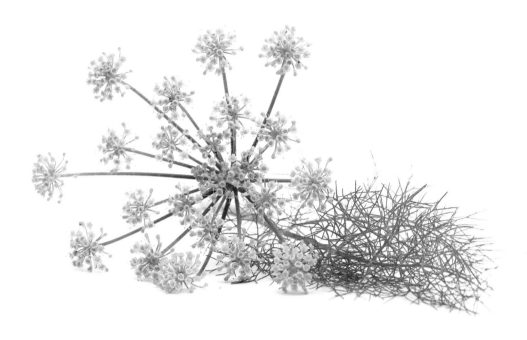

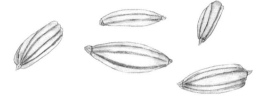

Note

Fennel seeds are rich in calcium, iron, magnesium, and manganese and may affect the absorption of any pharmaceutical drugs ingested. Do not ingest fennel seed essential oil, which is better used for mild facial issues (anti-aging and anti-wrinkles) or respiratory steams. As a phytoestrogen, she helps balance and stabilize hormone levels. Do not use when pregnant or if you have estrogen-dependent cancer. Fennel interacts with the antibiotic ciprofloxacin.

Make

Make a tea with ½ teaspoon crushed seeds to 1 cup (240 ml) boiling water and infuse for 15 minutes. The dose is ½ cup (120 ml) for adults, 2 to 3 teaspoons (10 to 15 ml) for infants and children. Make a strong decoction and simmer for 20 to 30 minutes with the lid on to capture her volatile oils. You want an oily film on the top of the water. Collect the pollen when the flowers are in bloom to add the aroma of licorice and curry to your Thai, Chinese, or Korean cooking.

Look-alikes

Fennel resembles poison hemlock (*Conium maculatum*), which is fatal if ingested.

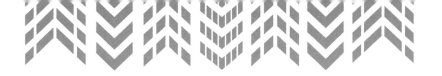

ECHINACEA

Echinacea angustifolia
Echinacea pallida
Echinacea purpurea

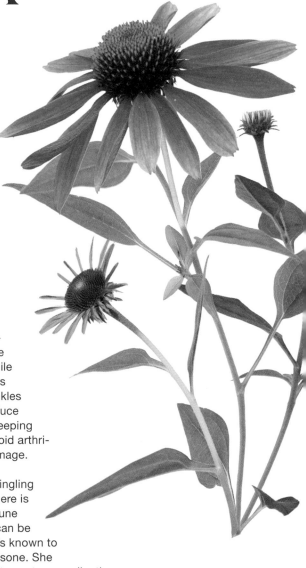

Beautiful *Echinacea angustifolia*. I am fascinated with her flower structure, as are pollinators, who love her for food. Growing flowers with our vegetables makes a vibrant garden. She was chewed by the Blackfoot to numb toothaches. The Dakota used her as an antidote for numerous poisonous bites. The Pawnee applied her juice for pain and burns. With *Echinacea pallida*, the Cheyanne decocted roots and leaves for rheumatism and arthritis. The Choctaw chewed *Echinacea purpurea* for cough medicine. The prairie settlers mixed the roots with animal feed for their horses and cows. Fresh leaves, stems, and flowers were given to horses for colic.

Echinacea is sweet and cooling to the body. She is not an antiviral but she stimulates the immune response as she raises white blood count, activating the T cells, which destroy foreign invaders. Combine her with reishi mushroom for Hashimoto's autoimmune inflammation. Echinacea contains chicoric acid, which inhibits hyaluronidase (an enzyme secreted by bacteria that breaks down hyaluronic acid), while decreasing the spread of bacteria and viruses. She contains hyaluronic acid to assist the skin in flexibility, reducing wrinkles and lines. She is helpful to promote wound healing and reduce scarring. She also works on the cartilage between joints, keeping them supple and viscous and therefore helpful for rheumatoid arthritis. We can apply her topically for prevention of UV sun damage.

You know your medicine is strong when you experience a tingling sensation on your tongue. Echinacea is best taken when there is a presence of pus anywhere on the body because the immune system is working hard to eliminate the waste. Echinacea can be called in to assist the body's defense system. *E. purpurea* is known to have the same anti-inflammatory effects as 100 mg of cortisone. She works as an endocannabinoid to moderate pain, gut mobility, motor coordination,

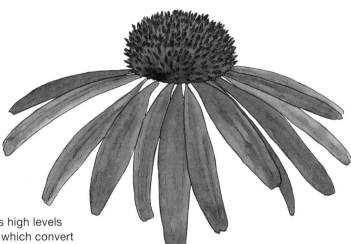

and eating challenges. She has high levels of seventeen hydroxysteroids, which convert androstenediones and testosterone back and forth, making her useful for men with low testosterone. Combine her with puncturevine (*Tribulus terrestris*) and pine pollen.

Collect the root in her third year of growth and tincture the whole plant. Leave the seed heads over winter to feed to our winged relatives.

Make

Make an herbal oil infusion with echinacea, calendula, dandelion root, and yarrow for dry eczema. For weeping eczema, blend with cleavers and Oregon grape root. If you are experiencing thick yellow phlegm, make an alcohol tincture and blend with Oregon grape root and usnea. It has been reported that, similar to a thuja alcohol tincture, echinacea helps alleviate ill effects of vaccinations. Make an oil infusion with mullein, fresh garlic, St. John's wort, and echinacea. When needed for acute inflammation or to treat severe conditions, use in combination with uva ursi.

Note

Large amounts can cause swelling. Avoid if you have allergies to the Asteraceae (daisy) family. Like grapefruit, echinacea can make pharmaceuticals either more effective or amplify side effects.

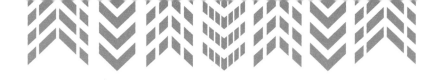

CANNABIS

Cannabis sativa
Cannabis indica
Cannabis ruderalis

Consider that our plants are teachers, alive with consciousness, living spirits. They are those who guide us when we sit, ask, and listen. Ganjah, cannabis's native name, has a centuries-long relationship with humanity around the world. Countless articles of cannabinoid research report her many benefits. Today, ganjah is seen as a commodity grown in greenhouses and bred for a high concentration of various chemical components.

She has been listed as medicine in countless herbalism books over the centuries, though not easily found in herbal materia medica today. We find accounts listed in Emperor Shen Nung's pharmacopeia dating back to 2800 BCE. She has a long spiritual relationship in India. Galen, a Roman and Greek physician (129–216 CE) reported the use of cannabis for therapeutic properties and mood enhancement. In 1841, William Brooke O'Shaughnessy, an Irish physician famous for his scientific work in pharmacology and chemistry, wrote about cannabis's benefits for children having convulsions. In 1936, the movie *Reefer Madness* depicted "marijuana" as a demonic, addictive drug causing mental illness and violence. In 1970, cannabis was listed in the Controlled Substances Act. The message was that cannabis had no accepted medical use and did have potential for misuse.

Various cannabinoids have been isolated since 1898. Dedi Meiri, one of the leading experts on ganjah, reports that there are over 550 strains of cannabis. It was fascinating to read the comments section from his TEDx talk posted in 2018 containing testimonies on the effectiveness of cannabis. The 1964 discovery of delta-9-tetrahydrocannabinol (THC) and cannabidiol (CBN) in cannabis eventually led to the discovery in 1988 of our endocannabinoid system. Cannabinoids found on the cannabis flower are similar to our own body's compounds that interact with our endocannabinoids system, the master regulator of homeostasis in the human body. This system governs and regulates sleep, eating, memory, and feelings of safety. In 1992, our own natural cannabinoid was revealed, anandamide (AEA), named from the Sanskrit word *ananda*, meaning "internal bliss." Cannabis can be a trickster and amplifies these experiences when we engage with her. We enjoy food more, she relaxes us to sleep, and she increases our forgetfulness. When used with a practice like meditation, she helps us find our center. Setting intentions to explore creativity, sexuality, and healing, ganjah brings a peaceful energy and folks are not typically violent under the influence.

Cannabis was listed in the United States Pharmacopeia from 1850 to 1937 for over a hundred illnesses. She was once administered for glaucoma and inflammation in ancient Egypt, and in 2012 she was been shown to alleviate schizophrenia comparable to synthetic antipsychotics. In 2017, cannabidiol (CBD), a phytocannabinoid, was shown to reduce seizures in childhood epilepsy. The cannabinoids interact with CD1 and CB2 receptors that treat a number of illnesses. This chemical bridge between the body and mind affects blood sugar, immune function, muscles, fat tissue, hormones, pain, dopamine, and our metabolic center.

Research abounds, but there can be many discrepancies based on numerous factors, such as dose, strain, metabolism, or simply the fact that ganjah is not your medicine. Some studies suggest that she will reinforce drug addiction or can be a treatment for drug addiction like nicotine. The endocannabinoid arachidonoyl ethanolamide (AEA) is reported by the National Library of Medicine to be a potent activator of tumor cell apoptosis (programs cell death). It is not clear how this mechanism works yet. AEA has a calming effect on stress-induced anxiety. Potential therapeutic

Make

For menstrual cramping, sciatica, and pelvic pain like endometriosis, make an infusion with her dried flowers and either coconut oil (which melts at 76°F [24.5°C]) or coconut butter (which melts at 93°F to 100°F [34°C to 37.8°C]). With all the different strains, how we respond is influenced by many factors. Consider doing research on suppositories. This application bypasses the liver, therefore not activating the brain with her "high." To activate the intoxicating components like THC, you need to heat to 300°F (150°C). This is known as decarboxylate.

continued on next page

endocannabinoid levels have been helpful for pain, depression, and psychiatric disorders. Many studies have demonstrated that AEA exerts an effect on the brain reward circuitry. We see that AEA levels are increased with the administration of morphine or heroin, which explains the addiction to these strong alkaloids. THC is the molecule that overactivates the parts of the brain that contain the highest amounts of receptors that stimulate the "high." Ganjah enhances and intoxicates us with her ability to expand our consciousness as she bonds with our serotonin, melatonin, and opioid receptors.

Cannabis is somewhat easy to grow as she will grow in a wide range of climates outdoors, although at the mercy of the weather. Indoors, in greenhouses, it is more precise. Check your local laws for guidance on whether or not, where, and how much you can legally grow. She needs lots of water, humidity, and nutrients from compost and compost teas.

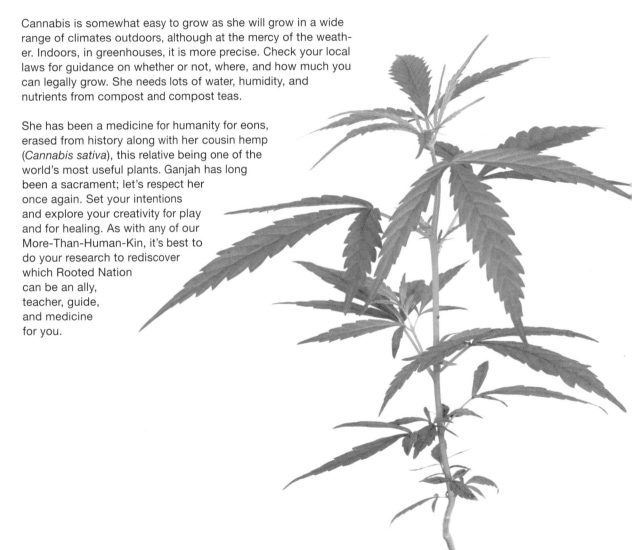

She has been a medicine for humanity for eons, erased from history along with her cousin hemp (*Cannabis sativa*), this relative being one of the world's most useful plants. Ganjah has long been a sacrament; let's respect her once again. Set your intentions and explore your creativity for play and for healing. As with any of our More-Than-Human-Kin, it's best to do your research to rediscover which Rooted Nation can be an ally, teacher, guide, and medicine for you.

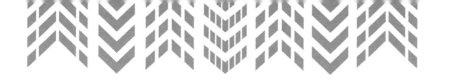

GOLDENROD

Solidago canadensis

According to the database Plants for a Future, there are no known hazards with goldenrod. A host and nectar plant for pollinators, this late-blooming hermaphrodite (contains both male and female flowers) hosts abundant blooms in the autumn months. She is beneficial for ladybugs, lacewings, and hoverflies.

Solidago virgaurea is the most clinically studied of the more than one hundred species we find. Goldenrod's Latin name, *solidago*, means "to make whole or heal," and she offers a safe and gentle remedy for urinary tract infections. As a strong diuretic that flushes out harmful bacteria, she may retain extra sodium in your body, which will affect high blood pressure. She is helpful for overactive bladders when combined with juniper berry and horsetail. She contains saponins that are antifungal for *Candida albicans*. The rutin helps support capillary frugality and the flavonoids of kaempferol and quercetin are known potent anticancer and anti-inflammatory agents.

Goldenrod prefers full sun to part shade and handles dry soil. Designing a garden with a succession of blooms from early spring to late fall benefits all our creatures. Goldenrod's bright yellow clusters of flowers appear on the top of tall woody stems from July to September, making her an excellent choice for late season blooms.

Make

Goldenrod is edible, so we can collect seeds for thickening soups. Remember to leave the stocks standing over winter so the seeds can be food for birds. Cook the leaves when young, and make a tea from all aerial parts of the plant. For ulcers and wounds, make a poultice with her flowers. She creates a mustard-orange botanical dye. Use the roots for boils.

Note

If you have allergies to latex, or have congestive heart disease, kidney disease, or are pregnant or breastfeeding, do not use goldenrod. It is not recommended for children under twelve.

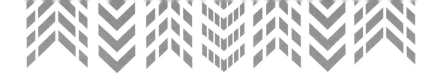

ROSE

Rosa rugosa
Rosa canina

Living in an urban landscape I am always on the lookout for spaces where I can collect medicines. In the small school that my daughters attended, planted along a chain link fence in the back alley are numerous gifts of *Rosa canina* rosehips. Rosehips are best collected after the first frost. Our winters are mild, so it may be very late in the season before we get a frost. I pay attention to the rains and collect her before the rosehips get too soft. Here on the West Coast various species of rose grow, like the Nootka rose (*Rosa nutkana*) and baldhip rose (*Rosa gymnocarpa*), both of which are a plentiful and important food source for the First Nations People. New shoots were collected in the spring and eaten raw or cooked. Infusions made with the root are used to wash the eyes or given for labor pain after birthing. A spit poultice can be made with the leaf for bee stings. Rosehips can be eaten fresh or dried and were made into dried berry cakes mixed with currants and elderberries and thickened with salmon eggs. These dried cakes were highly prized and used for trade. Be mindful of all the little hairs when eating fresh rosehips, as the hairs will make bowel movements itchy.

Dig up her root for a decoction to help cleanse the blood. Collect the leaves in the early spring before the flowers bloom and add them to salads or make an infusion to help with diarrhea, gastritis, stress, and infections. I take the fresh and dried petals that have fallen to Mother Earth. If we collect directly from the five-petaled flower, we are changing the outline of the flower's form, affecting bees' ability to find the flower. It is better to collect from the *Rosa rugosa*, as she has multiple flower petals. Lay out the petals overnight to let the water evaporate and then infuse them in honey. To help balance hormones, make a hydrosol with the petals. Rose petal tea is hydrating and can be applied as a skin wash to rebalance the pH and sebum on the skin and treat acne.

The rosehips are filled with bioflavonoids and make a great tonic for our hearts. Mineral-rich with abundant vitamins B and C, iron, and zinc, she stimulates the red blood cells. It has been reported that three rosehips are equivalent to the vitamin C in one orange. She is antispasmodic and antibacterial for the bladder and kidneys. She is helpful for hemorrhoids and varicose veins because she activates circulation. Rosehips also contain calcium, magnesium, phosphorus, potassium, proteins, selenium, and vitamins A and E. Rosehip seeds help get rid of intestinal parasites.

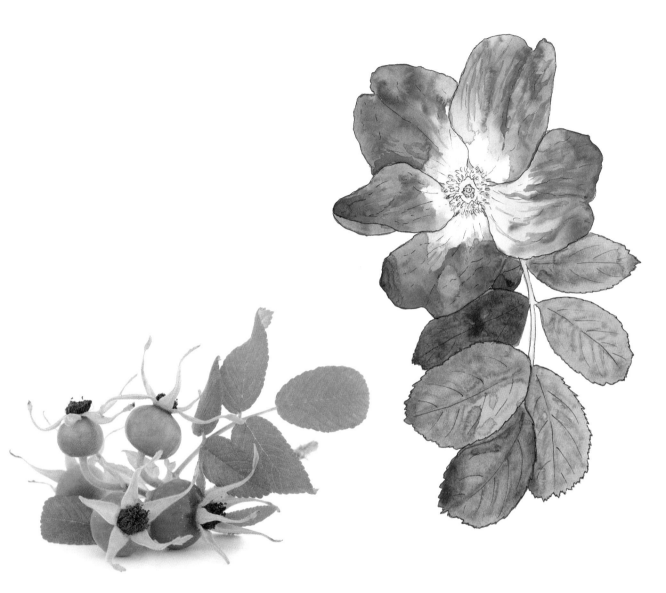

Musings

Under a microscope you can see that the structure of rose petals looks like puffy little duvet squares, a brilliant design of nature to efficiently hold her perfume.

Make

Use rosehips and rose petals to make syrup, gummies, jam, jelly, and ice cream. Steep a handful of crushed rosehips in hot water and strain (so as not to drink the hairs) for tea. Refill the pot with hot water up to three times for drinkable tea using the same rosehips.

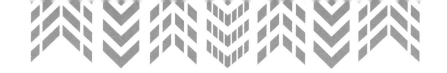

BURDOCK

Arctium lappa

A common herb native to Asia and Europe, today I rarely find burdock in our urban landscape. I love that her burr seeds are like Velcro and stick to everyone who passes by, migrating to different landscapes. Growing up through the cracks in sidewalks, she is strong and steady, rejuvenating chronic conditions and strengthening frail folk by bringing back their vigor. Burdock offers many gifts. She is high in iron and has an edible oxalic acid leaf and medicinal seeds and roots. It has also been said that burdock works on the brain, uterus, and prostate and can help with hair loss. Emotionally, burdock essences dispel our worry about the unknown, offering faith as we move forward.

Discovered by European allopathic doctors in the seventeenth century, burdock was introduced as an "alternative," a medicine that alters the system. In 1719, a London reporter on pharmacopeia noted that burdock was in much use among the country folk. *The Book of Herbal Wisdom: Using Plants as Medicines* by Matthew Wood has many accounts of various physicians and herbalists over the last three centuries who report successful accounts of healing with the administration of burdock.

Burdock cleanses the liver and kidneys by ridding the body of toxic waste. In the massive *King's American Dispensatory*, published in 1898, Felter and Lloyd reported on the action of the seeds, which are beneficial for dropsy, renal obstruction, and painful urination due to kidney stones. They wrote about its use for digestive disorders, bronchopulmonary irritation, psoriasis, eczema, and rheumatism. As a diaphoretic, she reduces fever. Today, burdock is prescribed as a blood purifier although she is much more than that.

Interchangeable and found in a wide range of climates, *Arctium lappa* and *Arctium minus* were previously known as *arcteion*, the Greek name for "bear plant." When she arrived on Turtle Island she was adopted by Indigenous People as a bear medicine. She is soothing to the mucous membranes, as the fats, oils, and starches are lubricating and coat inflamed tissue. All parts of burdock can be used for medicine. The fruit (seed), with her tingly, pungent flavor, activates our salivary glands, nourishing the digestive system. The seeds can be ingested for urinary calculi and have an influence on the kidneys. Many herbs with large leaves have a strong affinity to heal the skin and lungs. Use her leaf externally in salves or poultices. As a biennial with a deep taproot, it is best to collect her after the first season of her two-year biannual life cycle.

 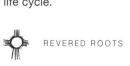

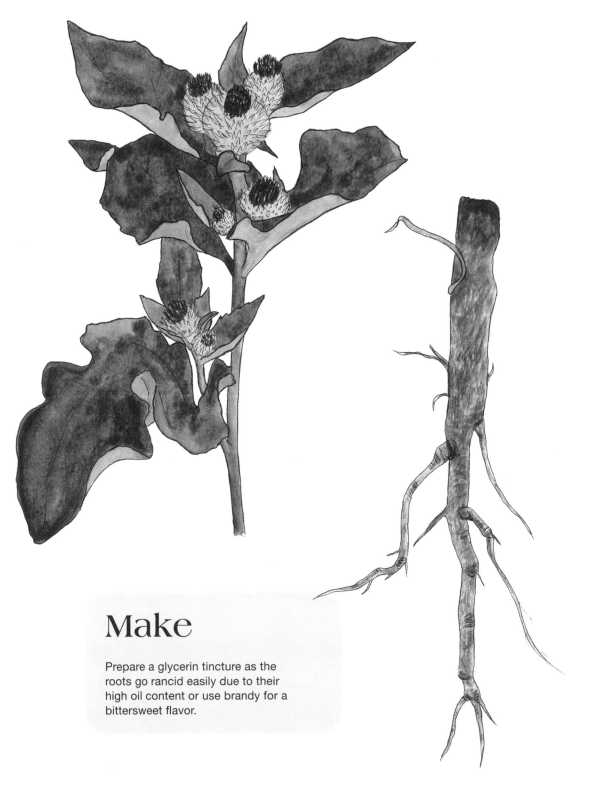

Make

Prepare a glycerin tincture as the roots go rancid easily due to their high oil content or use brandy for a bittersweet flavor.

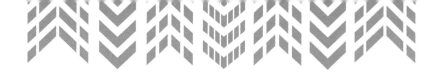

AMERICAN MAYAPPLE

Podophyllum peltatum

The Turtle Rescue League in Southbridge, Massachusetts, featured in the book *Of Time and Turtles: Mending the World, Shell by Shattered Shell*, written by Sy Montgomery and illustrated by Matt Patterson, explains how turtles have survived so long on Mother Earth. Their evolution is diverse, as is their contribution as a keystone species to other kin. I found it interesting to read in the book that the Asian mayapple's compound podophyllotoxin is a source for etoposide, powerful medication for inhibiting cell division and blocking the growth of tumors. Indeed, research in Europe is investigating mayapple's rhizome for the treatment of various forms of cancer.

Unfortunately, Asian mayapple is overharvested almost to the point of extinction. An effective substitute is the American mayapple, *Podophyllum peltatum*; however, she comes with the challenge of difficult propagation as biological digestion of the seeds needs to take place. This is why the box turtle (*Terrapene carolina*) is an important contributor to the plant's life cycle. Box turtles ingest and excrete mayapple seeds and act as a slow, mobile seed spreader. The germination rate for these "planted" seeds is low and seedlings are frequently unsuccessful, as they are often shaded out.

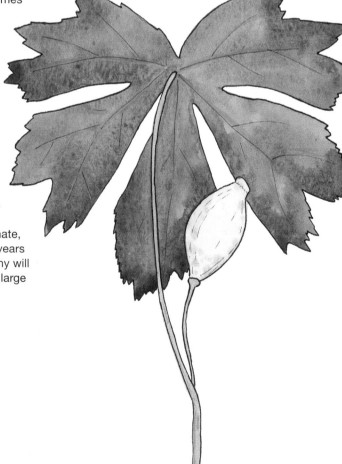

Successful pollination is also low, and few fruits are realized. The white flowers do offer pollen for native bees and bumblebees. Mayapple focuses her energy on the production of horizontal rhizomes for growing new offspring instead of putting energy into sexual production. Should a single seed germinate, a mayapple will not form a rhizome until she is five years old and flower when she is twelve years old. A colony will only grow 4 to 6 inches (10 to 15 cm) per year, so a large colony could be over a hundred years old.

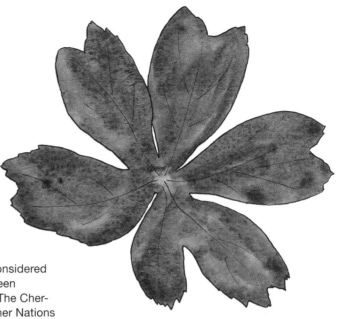

All of the plant, including the seeds, are considered toxic except for the ripe fruit, which has been described to taste like a Starburst candy. The Cherokee, Chippewa, Haudenosaunee, and other Nations ate mayapple fruits fresh and dried. It was used as a purgative, liver cleanser, and emetic. The Haudenosaunee decocted the leaves along with other plants, using the liquid to soak corn seeds before planting. The Cherokee used the root as an insecticide, soaking the corn to deter crows and insects. The list of applications by our Indigenous Nations and Tribes includes treatment for rheumatism, diarrhea, ulcers, sores, liver and bile challenges, hemorrhoids, headaches, whooping cough, and expelling worms. She is a diuretic and a laxative. In the early 1900s, American mayapple extract was one of the active ingredients for Carter's Liver Pills. Today you can purchase podophyllin, made from mayapple resin, for genital warts.

The overharvesting of plants worldwide is one of the many reasons Indigenous People are very careful about whom they share knowledge with. There is a deep love of protecting your kin and a veneration and humbling to Creator's gifts, which is alchemized through medicines and foods.

The box turtle, along with other Earth relatives like the white-footed mouse, gray squirrel, opossum, raccoon, grackle, fox, and black bear, are helpful seed dispersers.

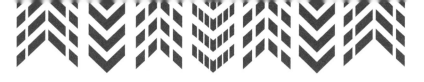

COTTONWOOD

Populus balsamifera ssp. *trichocarpa*
Populus deltoides
Populus balsamifera
Populus angustifolia
Populus alba
Populus fremontii

I am shown so much when I witness the bigger landscape and connect the strands that holds the ecosystem together. One summer while wandering along the riverbanks, I noticed little ponds flickering with small salmon called fry, growing to be ready for when the autumn rains overflow and sweep them to the ocean. Another time, I was surprised to see the base of a fallen cottonwood tree and observe the inner structure of this massive Rooted Nation. She looks like a giant sponge with the capacity to hold hundreds of gallons of water. The water is slowly released over the summer into those little ponds, nourishing the fry to help them survive the hot summer months. Cottonwood loves the water and we find her along waterways. She casts shadows and shade along the banks, cooling the temperature of the river, lakes, and streams. Along with many of our Rooted Nations, cottonwood is becoming endangered. All life connects in the web. When the temperature of the water rises, the salmon will not swim upstream to spawn.

Cottonwoods grow 6 feet (1.8 m) a year, to upward of 100 feet (30 m) tall. Eastern cottonwood (*Populus deltoides*) is found in the eastern United States and southern Canada; black cottonwood (*Populus balsamifera*) is found west of the Rocky Mountains; and Fremont cottonwood (*Populus fremontii*) is found from California east to Utah and from Arizona south into northwest Mexico. She is hardy in Zones 2 to 9, connecting all around Turtle Island. She has a very close relationship with our Indigenous Nations and is sometimes referred to as Balm of Gilead, a symbolic name reminding us of her power to soothe and heal.

You can collect the leaf buds from November to March. I like to gather after a windstorm, when Brother Wind has pruned her branches. Look for healthy buds without any black spots that may harbor mold. I find the buds from the upper wind-blown branches are twice the size of the little rice grain buds on the lower branches. The sticky aromatic resin is the medicine that is also collected by bees to make propolis. Cottonwood contains salicin, which converts to salicylate for pain-relieving properties. She is also antiseptic and helps with tissue regeneration, eczema, dry skin, diaper rash, and sunburns. Her inner bark was a survival food when needed, as it is full of vitamins and is a blood cleanser. Only the female cottonwood produces the fluffy, cotton-laden seeds, which can cause reactions in some folks. Her leaves have flat stems that shimmer, wave, and dance with Brother Wind.

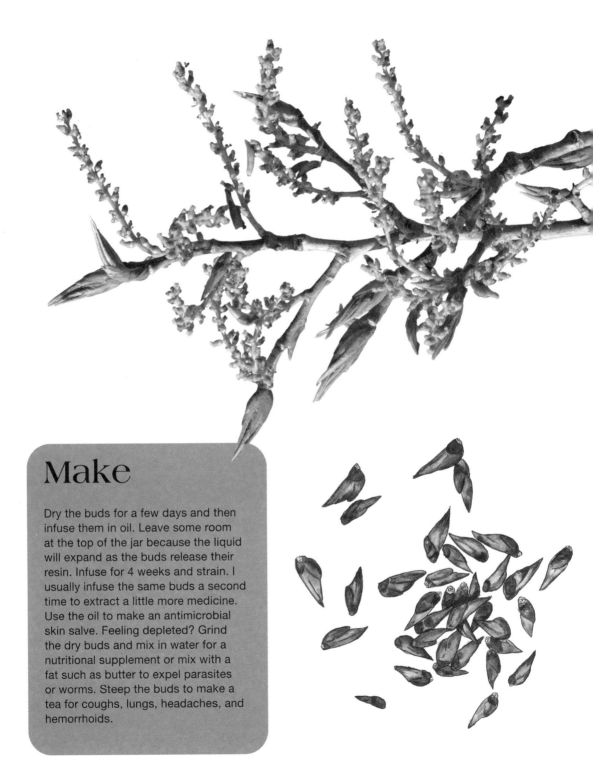

Make

Dry the buds for a few days and then infuse them in oil. Leave some room at the top of the jar because the liquid will expand as the buds release their resin. Infuse for 4 weeks and strain. I usually infuse the same buds a second time to extract a little more medicine. Use the oil to make an antimicrobial skin salve. Feeling depleted? Grind the dry buds and mix in water for a nutritional supplement or mix with a fat such as butter to expel parasites or worms. Steep the buds to make a tea for coughs, lungs, headaches, and hemorrhoids.

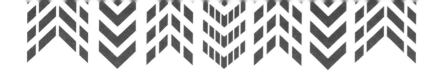

MAPLE

Acer saccharum

Maple has a long history as a food and medicine. Our Indigenous Nations celebrated and held ceremony to honor maple's gift through sacred dances, offerings of tobacco, sugar maple festivals, and community socials. The hardwood deciduous forest of the "maple belt," containing red, black, and sugar maples, is found in Ontario, Quebec, New Brunswick, Nova Scotia, Prince Edward Island, New England, and the Midwest. It is the homeland of our Indigenous Nations, who tapped the sugar maple in the late winter and early spring months. She is the "leader" tree, the first to wake up when the temperature rises above freezing during the day and drops below freezing at night. When the temperature fluctuates, the sugar sap starts to flow. The amazing process of maple syrup has sustained Indigenous People for thousands of years.

Among many Nations and Tribes, matrilineal lines passed on "ownership" of the maple groves. Thousands of handmade birch baskets made to collect the sap water were sewn with thin spruce roots and sealed with pine pitch. The baskets were set out overnight and the light water was skimmed off in the morning. The collected sap was cooked in carved-out logs using hot rocks to bring the sap to a boil. The women tended the fire to heat the rocks and maintained the sap at a low rolling boil. The heated stones made sure the maple sap was not over- or undercooked. The maple syrup was then poured into *mokuks*, tight birch bark boxes sewn together with strips of elm roots. The sugar would crystalize into sugar cakes weighing upwards of 30 pounds (13.5 kg), which were used for trade, curing meats, and as a sweetener.

When the settlers arrived in the seventeenth century, they cleared huge swaths of land, pushing Indigenous People away from their close interconnection to the land and their way of life. In 1876, the Indian Act in Canada forced resettlement and kept Indigenous Nations from their maple ceremonies and festivals. Today, many Nations are reclaiming this relationship to share in maple's many life-giving gifts again.

Maple syrup, dark blackstrap molasses, and raw honey all show antioxidant activity with their phenolic compounds. These compounds reduce free radical damage and the inflammation that

 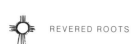

contributes to many chronic diseases. The darker maple syrup contains even more beneficial antioxidants, such as benzoic, gallic and cinnamic acids, and the flavonoids catechin, epicatechin, rutin, and quercetin. She offers inflammation-taming red polyphenols, which are helpful in preventing arthritis, irritable bowel syndrome, and heart disease. Her plant-based compounds reduce oxidative stress known to age us quicker and impact our immune system.

Maple syrup provides zinc, which helps combat illness and boosts immunity by increasing white blood cells; manganese, which affects our fat and carbohydrate metabolism; calcium; and potassium.

Researcher Nathalie Tufenkji observed that when maple syrup extracts were administered with the antibiotics ciprofloxacin and carbenicillin, it increased the permeability of the bacteria cell walls, allowing the antibiotics to be 90 percent more effective. In animal studies, maple syrup lowered cholesterol in mice. Other studies show benefits for neurodegenerative diseases.

Make

Prepare a hydrating and calming skin mask with maple syrup, yogurt, rolled oats, and raw honey.

The time of maple sap collecting is known as *Ziisbaakdoke Dbik Giizis*, the Sugar Moon or Maple Moon in Ojibwe. *Sinzibuckwud* is an Algonquin word for "drawn from the wood."

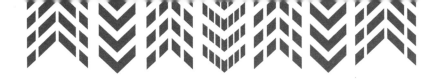

JUNIPER BERRIES

Juniperus communis

Ten years ago, I was teaching gardening to the children at one of the local schools and I was grateful to discover a native juniper tree growing in the landscape. Recently, I stopped by the school to find that she is dying. Thankfully, she offered some of her berries with her seeds inside to regenerate a new generation. Juniper berries take around three years to mature and ripen, and they contain chromium, cobalt, iron, magnesium, manganese, niacin, phosphorus, potassium, riboflavin, selenium, sodium, thiamine, and protein.

Juniper can be used topically for various skin conditions. Gather her needles any time of the year to infuse in oil for sore muscles and pain. She is a diuretic, an antiseptic for urinary infections, and anti-inflammatory. She is helpful for gout and nerve pain like sciatica, is a digestive, relieves gas, and lowers blood pressure. She purifies the blood, removing acids and waste.

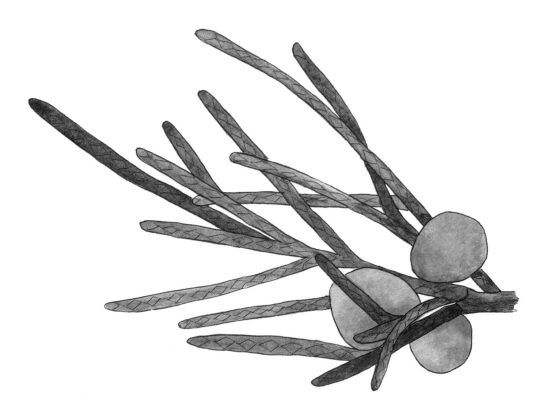

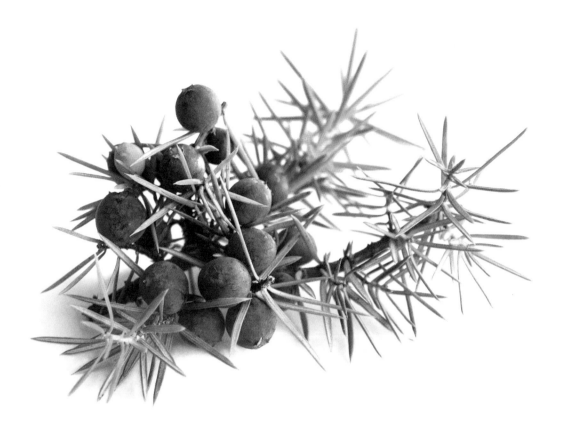

Make

Add juniper needles to saunas or for steaming when feeling congested. Prepare a juniper butter by blending 8 berries with 1 cup (225 g) butter, diced onion, a few cloves of minced garlic, and 2 to 3 tablespoons (30 to 45 ml) seed oil. Serve with meat dishes or atop fresh bread. Store the butter in the fridge. Make juniper tea, a poultice, or an infused oil for creams and salves. Apply to your body before you get in the bath.

Note

The species *Juniperus communis* is typically used for flavoring and made into gin. Other varieties like *Juniperus sabina* and *Juniperus oxycedrus* are toxic. Collect juniper berries from plants that you can positively identify. Consume in small amounts as they may irritate your kidneys.

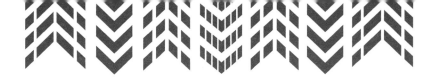

USNEA

Usnea barbata
Usnea longissima
Usnea californica

In 2018, I walked for four days in the jungle in the Amazon basin and as we were departing I finally found a plant I could identify! My dear brother Flavio's mother shared that they administered usnea medicine to stop the bleeding during childbirth, and the same is done up here in the North.
I only gather her after a windstorm, when she is "given" to Mother Earth versus "taken" from her home in the branches of the Rooted Nations.
I dose myself with fresh plant tincture when I have an infection or need an herbal antibiotic. Usnea is classified as a lichen, an interconnected relationship between an algae (the food) and a fungi (the structure housing the algae). She is helpful for weight loss, pain, fever, wound healing, and phlegm.

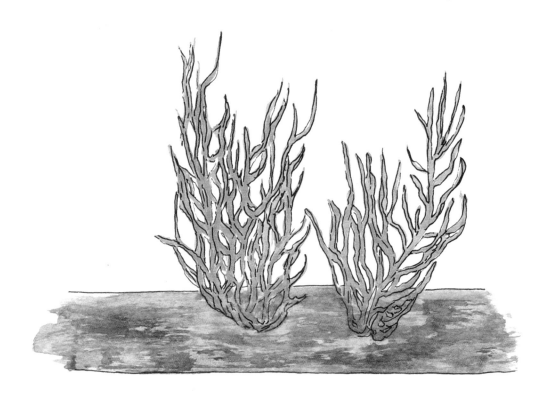

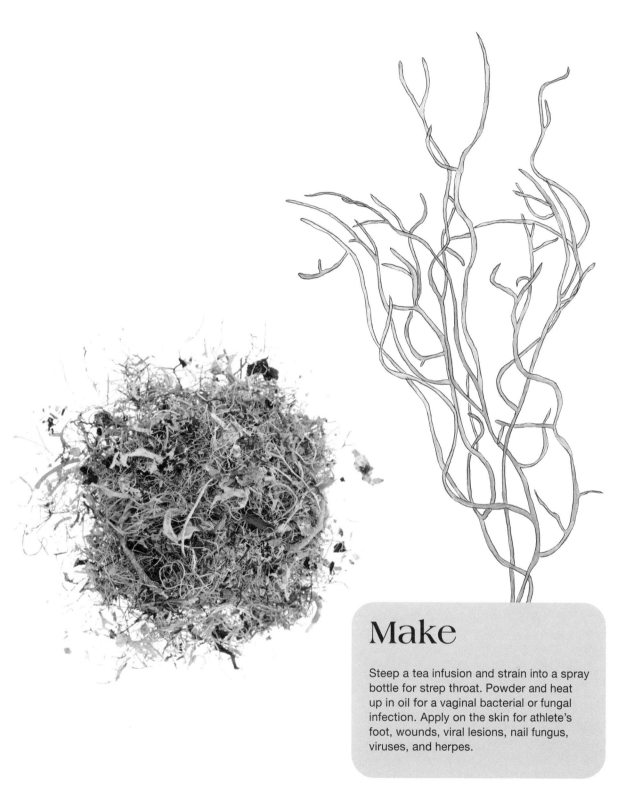

Make

Steep a tea infusion and strain into a spray bottle for strep throat. Powder and heat up in oil for a vaginal bacterial or fungal infection. Apply on the skin for athlete's foot, wounds, viral lesions, nail fungus, viruses, and herpes.

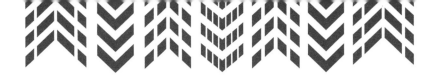

CRESS

Barbarea verna
Barbarea vulgaris

Cress, *Barbarea*, is a very early, spring green who graces us with her tastiness and spiciness. She is one of the oldest cultivated leaf vegetables. At one time she was collected on December 4th to honor Saint Barbara's Day. Eaten by ducks, muskrats, and deer, she has a long history of medicinal uses during Roman times. The cresses were in high favor around 1776, for their warm, bitter taste and antiscorbutic and diuretic properties. This little green was the only fresh vegetable available to the early settlers during the colder parts of the year. High in vitamins A and C, she was known as "scurvy grass." She was used as a mild stimulant, a source of phytochemicals, an expectorant, a digestive, and a diuretic. In Iran, research revealed her antioxidant properties, lowering cholesterol and triglycerides. In the United States research shows promise for treating or preventing cancer.

We can gather land cress (*Barbarea verna* or *B. vulgaris*) and two similar species: watercress (*Nasturtium officinale*) and garden cress (*Lepidium sativum*). Land cress has various other names, including American cress, dryland cress, cassabully, winter cress, creasy greens, and highland creasy. In the Pacific Northwest, we also find bittercress, *Cardamine oligosperma*. In your area you might gather *Cardamine bulbosa* (bulbous bittercress), *C. pensylvanica* (Pennsylvania bittercress), or *Arabis alpina* (alpine rock cress). We do have a native cress, *Barbarea orthoceras*, but according to the USDA Plants Database, it has become quite rare.

Land cress is easier to grow than watercress, is rich in nutrients such as calcium and iron, and has a crisp, strong peppery flavor, adding depth to our salads. Ask for her by using her botanical name when purchasing seeds. *Vulgaris* refers to "common" and *verna* refers to "spring." Both species of land cress look alike, are grown around the same time, and can be collected as food. Planted in cool, moist soil with some shade, this perennial member of the mustard family will go to flower and seeds in hot weather. We can find cress in late winter and early spring before any other greens. She is hardy through mild freezing temperatures and then she grows again in the fall. When the weather is still cold, collect either the leaf or the whole plant when she is 4 inches (10 cm) tall. Once the energy goes into the blooms and seeds, her peppery flavor becomes tough and bitter. Many foragers recommend parboiling the leaves for 1 minute prior to sautéing with olive oil, garlic, and a squeeze of lemon. The cress with yellow flowers is also edible and can be dried to make a naturally sweet tea.

 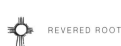

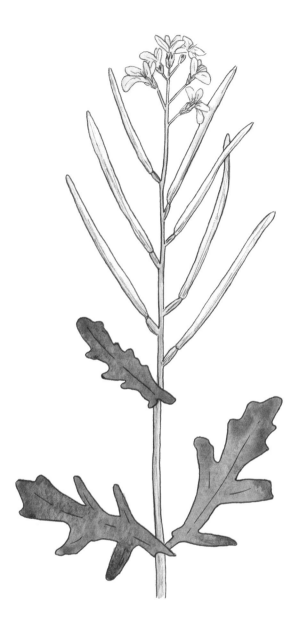

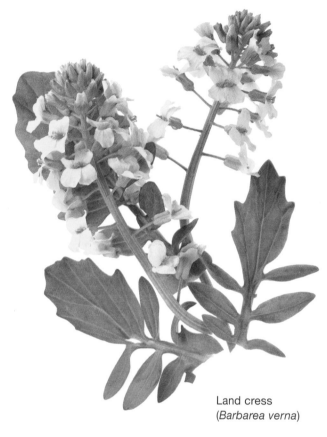

Land cress
(*Barbarea verna*)

Make

Eat cress while in season, cooking the leaves like spinach.

Note

Cress may cause cystitis for some folks. Do not consume if you have a delicate stomach or suffer from acidosis or heartburn. Excessive consumption may lead to kidney problems. Avoid while pregnant or breastfeeding.

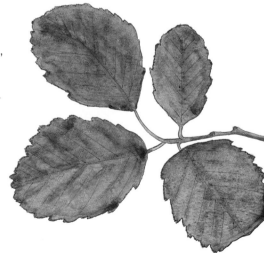

ALDER

Alnus rubra
Alnus incana
Alnus rhombifolia

Another of many Rooted Nations, Alder has been in an interconnected relationship with many Nations and Tribes across Turtle Island. The Nuxalk People of the Northwest Pacific Coast used the cones of *Alnus incana*, mountain alder, for medicine. The Chippewa infused the bark for anemia or made a decoction of the root and powdered bumblebees for difficult labor. The Woodland Cree made a decoction of the inner bark to wash the eyes. The Ojibwe used her as an astringent and coagulant when a person had bloody stools. The wood charcoal was mixed with pitch to seal canoe seams. The Tete-de-Boule, known as the Atikamekw People of Quebec, made yellow dye with her inner bark.

The Algonquin People mixed the root bark of the speckled alder (*Alnus incana* ssp. *rugosa*) with molasses for toothaches and used it as a laxative and an emetic. The Gitksan People used the thin leaf alder (*Alnus incana* ssp. *tenuifolia*) to make a diuretic with bark shavings and also made a gonorrhea treatment with the catkins. The Woodland Cree used the reddish orange dye of red alder to color porcupine quills. The Pomo People of Mendocino, California, dried the bark of white alder (*Alnus rhombifolia*) to make a decoction for diarrhea and as a blood purifier; they also made a poultice of her dried wood for burns. The Inuktitut-speaking people of the Arctic poulticed leaves of American green alder (*Alnus viridis* ssp. *crispa*) and burned the wood to inhale for rheumatism. The bark was also soaked to make a rusty orange dye to color tanned skins. Red alder (*Alnus rubra*) was used as medicine, food, dye, fiber, baskets, cradleboards, rattles, and ceremonial items like masks and feast bowls. Red alder wood is soft until hardened by water, which the Norse People from the Scandinavian countries used to build boats.

One of our local alders is the red alder, *Alnus rubra*. My brother-in-law, Rod, introduced me to her and shared that red alder only lived for about forty years. She is a pioneer tree, a "community builder" that is fast growing in areas that have been devastated by wildfires, logging, and other disasters. Alders heal damaged ecosystems by rebuilding the soil. Her extensive fibrous root system forms a symbiotic relationship with actinomycetes, nitrogen-fixing bacteria. Filamentous bacteria form nodules on the alder's root hairs, and these nodules provide a home for the bacteria that remove the atmospheric nitrogen produced. This promotes the growth of other species that help regenerate the land.

Growing upward of 100 feet (30 m), alder prefers wet forests and waterways. She works with her community to form groves

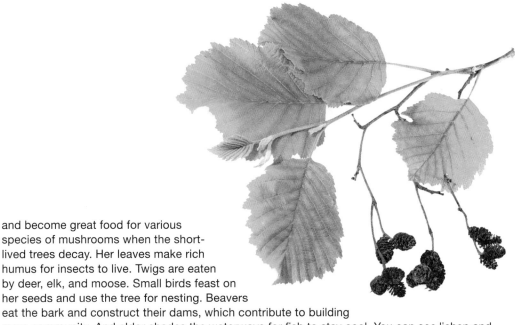

and become great food for various species of mushrooms when the short-lived trees decay. Her leaves make rich humus for insects to live. Twigs are eaten by deer, elk, and moose. Small birds feast on her seeds and use the tree for nesting. Beavers eat the bark and construct their dams, which contribute to building more community. And alder shades the waterways for fish to stay cool. You can see lichen and moss growing with her. Her leaves are toothed and pointed at the tip and base and she has both male catkins and female cones that resemble small brown pine cones.

Alder's essence communicates spiritual strength, fortitude, and resilience. She moves and balances body fluids and is astringent, cooling, and drying. Known as a skin healer, she reduces swelling. She is also used for chronic conditions when patterns of sluggishness are present. She is antiviral, antifungal, and antipathogenic. Use red alder for sore joints, flus and colds, kidney infections, and as a bitter for indigestion. Suck on the fresh, green male catkins or female green cones as a lozenge for sore throats.

Look-alikes

Here on the West Coast a similar look-alike is cascara sagrada (*Frangularia purshiana*).

Note

Use for short periods of time as too much may make you vomit, unless you need an emetic. Red alder teas are not recommended as the water draws out lots of tannins, impairing digestion.

Make

Make an alcohol tincture with one part dried bark, dried green female cones, and fresh catkins to five parts alcohol. Prepare an oil infusion with freshly dried twigs, leaf buds, and catkins. Add red alder to a footbath to strengthen your feet. Gargle with infused alder tea for canker sores or infected gums.

Other nitrogen-fixing plants are found in the legume family, like alfalfa, lupins, peanuts, rooibos, vetch, clover, and soybeans.

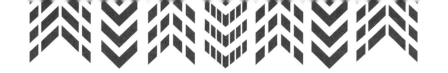

WINTERGREEN

Gaultheria procumbens

Wintergreen's cousin, *Gaultheria shallon*, known as salal, grows here on the West Coast and provides a deep purple berry gift full of omega-3s to feed our brains. Wintergreen, too, gifts us with her berry; however, the red berry is quite different, with its zingy, cool, wintergreen flavor, a flavor that is familiar in toothpaste or chewing gum.

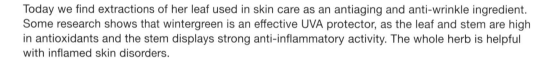

As a polyphenolic-rich medicine and food, wintergreen's ethnopharmacology provides insight into her anti-inflammatory, antioxidant, and antimicrobial properties. The Haudenosaunee infused wintergreen for cold remedies, making poultices of the whole plant to apply to the chest or infusing leaves for stomachaches. The Cherokee used wintergreen and trailing arbutus for chronic indigestion and chewed the leaves for tender gums. The Chippewa made a decoction in the spring and fall to cleanse the blood. The Lenape combined wintergreen with poke root, mullein leaves, wild cherry, and black cohosh for a treatment for rheumatism and made a tea as a tonic. The Shinnecock Tribe prepared wintergreen infusions for kidney troubles.

Today we find extractions of her leaf used in skin care as an antiaging and anti-wrinkle ingredient. Some research shows that wintergreen is an effective UVA protector, as the leaf and stem are high in antioxidants and the stem displays strong anti-inflammatory activity. The whole herb is helpful with inflamed skin disorders.

In the marketplace, the essential oil of wintergreen is found in over-the-counter products such as deep heating creams for muscle and joint pain relief and in Chinese medicinal liniments. The essential oil is mainly comprised of methyl salicylate, which is structurally similar to acetylsalicylic acid, which we find in aspirin.

Some folks have allergies or sensitives to salicylates. Overuse of salicylate can lead to salicylism, with symptoms of dizziness, nausea, vomiting, tinnitus, hyperventilation, and changes in mental status that could lead to coma and then death. A 2013 study showed oral hygiene benefits of wintergreen's essential oil on dental cavities caused by the pathogen *Streptococcus mutans*. She has antimicrobial effects on other pathogens as well, including *Candida albicans, Streptococcus sanguis, Streptococcus pyogenes, Pseudomonas aeruginosa*, and *Staphylococcus aureus*.

Wintergreen is a potent ally and as such we need to be mindful of potential side effects from repeated applications. Methyl salicylate is rapidly absorbed through the gastrointestinal tract and through dermal application. One drop of wintergreen essential oil is equivalent to 81 mg of baby aspirin. Grow some wintergreen, eat some berries, make a tea, and respect our Rooted Nations' potent gifts.

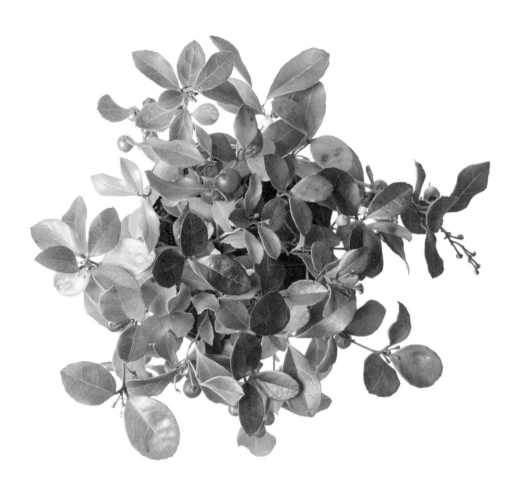

Musings

It's best practice to diversify your pain medication. Ask yourself what the root cause of the pain is. Is your body saying "no" to some activity or way of being that is not serving you?

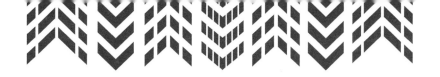

WITCH HAZEL

Hamamelis virginiana

In the month of January, while out walking around, we may be blessed to discover witch hazel, with her wild yellow, orange, or red spidery flowers. Her fragrant spicy odor attracts noctuid or owlet moths, native bees, and a diversity of other flying insects. She is host to the spring azure butterfly and food for our four-legged and winged relatives, like grouse and pheasant. Witch hazel has been a folk and Indigenous medicine for a very long time due to her natural astringent and antiseptic qualities. The Mamaceqtaw Tribe made sacred beads from the seeds for their medicine ceremonies. Early settlers used her forked crooked branches to dowse for underground water.

Topically, witch hazel's properties help relieve pain and irritation from acne, varicose veins, hemorrhoids, dandruff, stretch marks, wounds, and insect and spider bites. Do not use on your skin if you are experiencing burning, stinging, or flushing symptoms. Rich in hamamelitannin, witch hazel is known to inhibit pathogenic bacteria, offer probiotic bacteria help to foster a balanced microbiome, and maintain homeostasis gut health. The challenge for the gut biome is to have more probiotic bacteria versus the pathogenic bacteria that can be influenced by stressors and nutritional variants. *Lactobacillus plantarum* are commonly digested through fermented foods and found in the gastrointestinal tract. Imbalances in the gut lead to various digestive, dietary, metabolic, and mental health issues. The gastrointestinal tract contains such a diverse biome that both good and not-so-good bacteria can be disrupted by many factors. Long-term use of antibiotics has been known to destroy a balanced microflora, giving way to antibiotic-resistant strains and bacterial overgrowth, like the sometimes deadly *Clostridium difficile*.

Witch hazel likes moist sites on east- and north-facing slopes where she is food for white-tailed deer, beavers, and rabbits. Once her flower is pollinated, she will eventually eject and explode out her seeds up to 12 feet (3.6 m). Harvest the suckers for the bark and twigs that are growing up from the base of the small 20-foot (6 m) tree during the winter season.

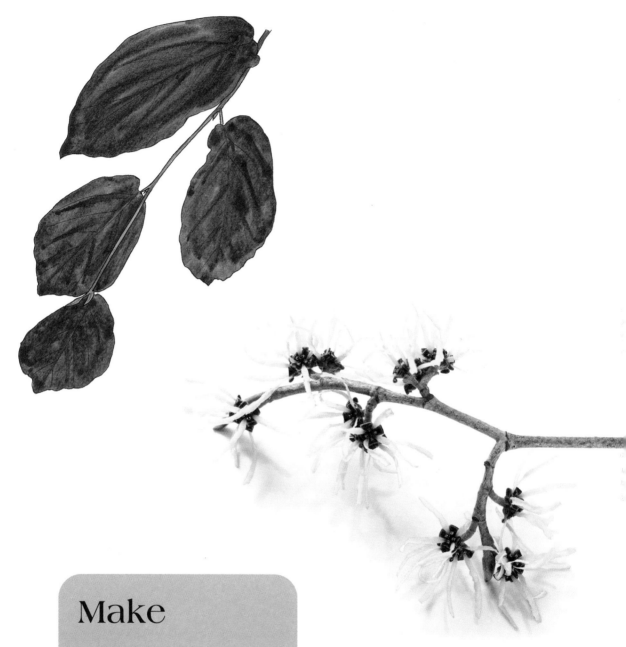

Make

Prepare a witch hazel hydrosol with peeled bark and small twigs. Add 1 cup (240 ml) alcohol when simmering. The timing depends on the density of the herb; it could take anywhere from 45 minutes to 1½ hours to steam distill witch hazel's gifts. Strain and label, and store in the fridge to preserve longer.

We are reminded that the interconnected relationship goes beyond people and plants. Our Rooted Nations not only provide food and medicine, gifts of beauty, and teachings, they also participate and contribute to our spiritual practices.

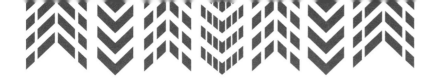

YUCCA

Yucca baccata

My parents had a yucca growing on the side of my childhood home. Her basal rosette shape with evergreen, sharply pointed leaves, often with white curling hairs, was striking to witness. Even more impressive, yucca's mass of creamy white-green flowers form on a regal, tall stalk that can grow up to 10 feet (3 m). She is found in a variety of mixed environments, from grasslands to deserts to here on the West Coast. All yucca species depend on pollination from a nocturnal yucca moth (*Tegeticula yuccasella*), as each variety of this moth adapts to each species of yucca.

Many Tribes across Turtle Island have a deep, long-standing, engaged, and dynamic interconnection with yucca. The Choctaw Nation used *Yucca aloifolia* root, boiled and mashed, to mix with animal grease or tallow for a skin salve. The Apache used *Yucca angustissima* for snake and insect bites. The Hopi baked the fruit with lamb's quarter leaf and ate them with corn dumplings. *Yucca baccata* fruit was eaten by many Tribes, made into beverages, or dried for winter use. The Pima of Gila River made them into sweets. The Apache made cordage with the leaf and stalk. Many Tribes made footwear with the leaf, weaving patterns so others could identify whose family was traveling through. She was woven into mats, rugs, bedding, sifters, and baskets. Dried leaves were boiled with gums, hardened, powdered, and mixed with water to waterproof baskets. *Yucca elata* was used in various ceremonies, as were some other yucca species.

A 2024 medical review reports yucca's many benefits in animal experiments. In studies with diabetic rats, Mojave yucca (*Y. schidigera*) reduced glucose levels, increased insulin, improved cholesterol, and showed antioxidant effects. Yucca's active constituents exert anti-inflammatory, antimicrobial, and antioxidant activity, with a positive impact on animal fertility. She has been reported to be beneficial for migraines, hypertension, high cholesterol, arthritis, and colitis. Mojave yucca has a bittersweet taste and foams when added to water and shaken. The extract is used commercially as a foaming agent found in flavorings and beverages. The roots and flowers have the steroidal glycosides of sapogenin, sarsasapogenin,

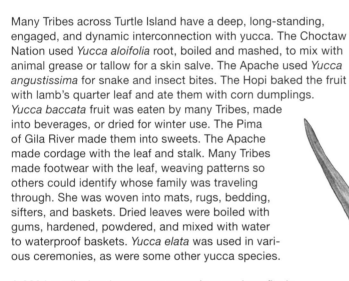

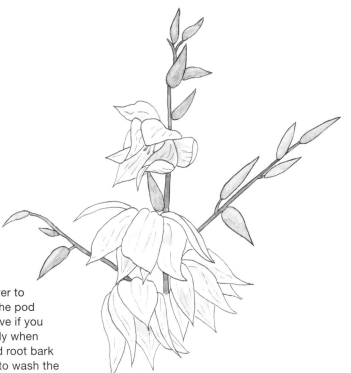

tigogenin, furostanol, and spirostanol. Antiviral activity was reported with *Yucca gloriosa*, making her helpful for herpes simplex viruses type 1 and 2.

All species are edible. Collect the flower to eat fresh, dried, steamed, or boiled. The pod offers a sweet fruit that is mildly laxative if you eat too much. The seed pods are ready when they are caramel in color. The root and root bark are full of saponins that make a soap to wash the hair, body, and clothes.

Note

Saponins are poisonous to other life forms and mostly nontoxic to us when taken orally. Do not use for long periods of time. Yucca root found in grocery stores is actually cassava root (*Manihot esculenta*) and is a completely different species.

Make

Prepare a soup with onion, garlic, squash, and yucca flowers. Scoop out the seeds from the pod, then roast, dry, and pound them into edible cakes.

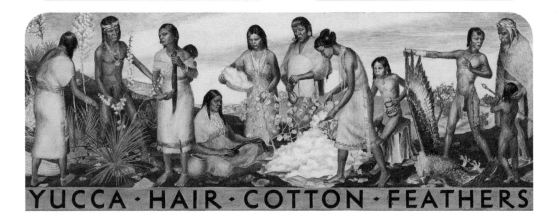

YUCCA · HAIR · COTTON · FEATHERS

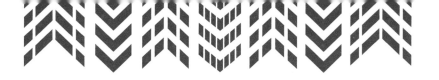

RED OSIER DOGWOOD

Cornus sericea

Miskwaabiimizh in Anishinaabe, red osier dogwood is a common name for several species. The Cherokee People used flowering dogwood (*Cornus florida*) as a medicine to "sweat off the flu." The Algonquin mixed a small herb, bunchberry dogwood (*Cornus canadensis*) with other plants for menstrual spasms, to strengthen the uterine muscle, and to help remove the endometrial lining. They also ate the berries as a snack food. The Hoh People used Pacific dogwood (*Cornus nuttallii*) as medicine, the berries for ceremony, and smoked the leaves. Joseph Pitawanakwat, an Anishinaabe plant medicine educator, shares stories of how the women in northern communities drink dried and powdered pith tea while in labor to help with the pain. He also reports that the medicine inhibits cell growth and reabsorbs calcium for folks suffering with rheumatoid arthritis. Dogwood can be used as an alternative to willow if you have allergies to salicin. The bark of all members of the *Cornus* genus, except bunchberry, has been known as a substitute for quinine to increase circulation, strengthen the walls of the lower intestine, and clean out the stomach.

Red osier dogwood has been used for building sweat lodges. When her flexible branches touch Mother Earth, she will grow another clone. Her bright red bark stands out in the winter months, when it is best to collect her wood, although you can collect in any season. Within a week after gathering, use a potato peeler to remove the outer bark, then scrape the inner bark and pith. After a week she will dry out and be more difficult to peel, as she becomes a very hard wood once dried. Red osier prefers cool, wet areas. Her white flowers are visible at night and make a relaxing, calming tea. Her leaf is a nursery for spring azure butterflies (*Celastrina ladon*) and deer, moose, rabbits, and chipmunks love to browse on her winter twigs. The berries ripen in August and will stay on the tree until the winter. Cardinals, starlings, grosbeaks, cedar waxwings, and grackles have been witnessed feasting on the fermented berries, flying around inebriated.

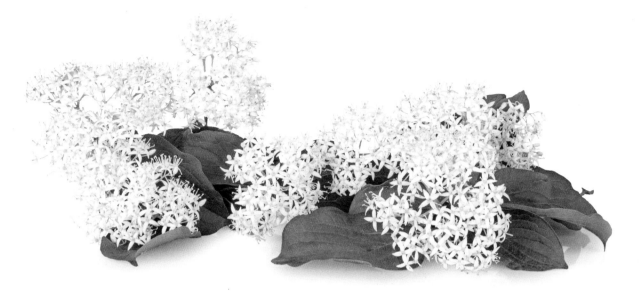

Note

Do not use when pregnant. You may experience some diarrhea.

Make

Dogwood tea can help with the build-up of acids aggravated by excessive sugar, insulin, and stress. Prepare tea with ½ ounce (10 to 15 g) of herb in 1 gallon (3.8 L) water. Drink 2 to 3 cups (480 to 720 ml) daily and you may notice a big difference within 8 months. Soak a cloth in the tea, freeze, and offer to teething babies.

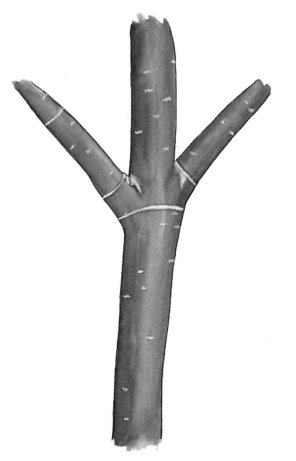

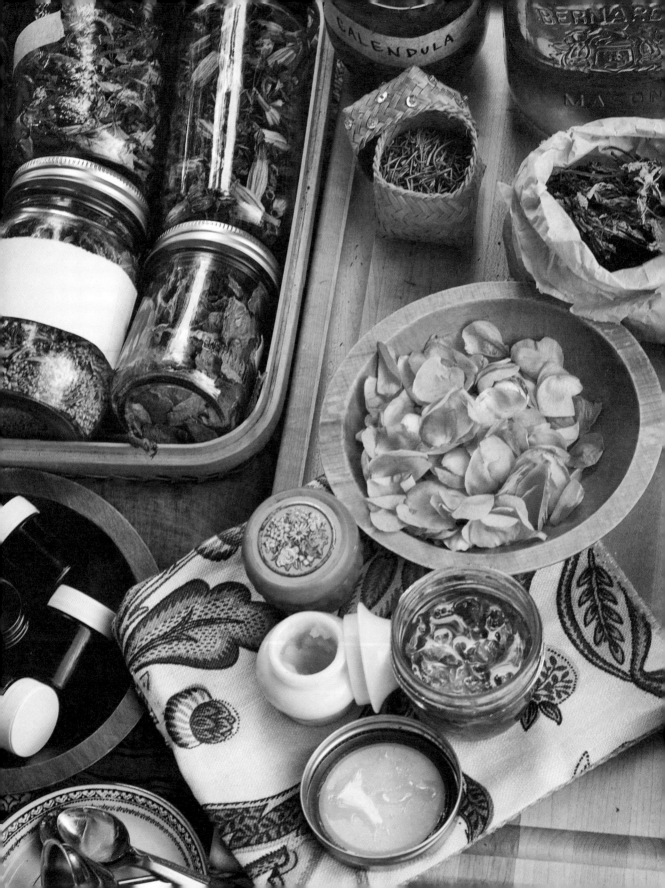

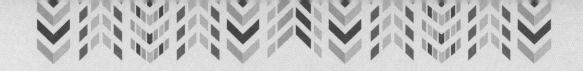

PART III

The Art of Medicine Making

Good Practices
Here are some suggestions to keep in mind before, during, and after you gather medicines.

1. Ask permission from our Rooted Nations before you collect, and leave an offering of prayers and gratitude. In our Indigenous practices we will leave sacred medicine.

2. Gather your tools and ensure they are clean and dry.

3. Take only what you need and will use in a season or year.

4. Gather after the morning dew so that what you collect is dry and less susceptible to mold.

5. Collect and place in paper bags, as plastic will make your herbs sweat.

6. Use glass and wooden utensils, as plastic leaches and metal sterilizes.

7. Seal your bottles well as air oxidizes and evaporates alcohol.

8. Choose organic, local, and quality products for your medicines; it makes a difference.

9. Label, with the herb name, date collected and where, and the moon phase if you'd like.

10. Store your medicines in dark glass, in a cool area and away from direct sunlight and heat.

11. To give back to Mother Earth, compost your herbs after you strain out the medicines.

12. Be creative about how you use your medicines, such as in a tea or tincture, in soups and stews, and in your bath.

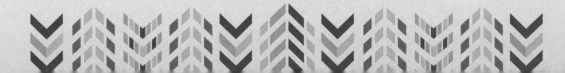

Dosages

It is a journey to determine what dosage will work best for you. Our physiology, age, temperament, the conditions we may be experiencing, level of stress, how we digest, and whether we are pregnant or lactating can all affect the dose. Start slow, pay attention, and make notes. If something feels off, stop taking the medicine. Test out the herb by rubbing it on the inner skin of your arm and see whether you have any reaction. If you are allergic to one plant in a particular family, then you will most likely be allergic to other plants in the same family. Be mindful of interactions with pharmaceuticals, whether prescribed or over-the-counter medications. Ask for support from a qualified practitioner of herbal medicine if you have serious medical conditions.

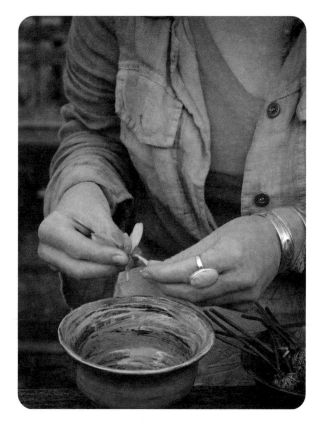

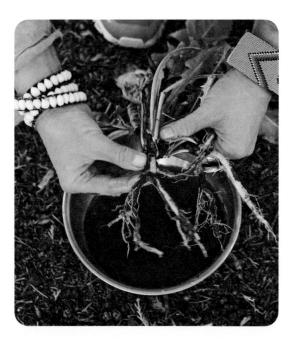

Medicine Making

Medicinal preparation depends upon which biochemical agent of the herb is extracted and the qualities that it influences in our body. Some medicines work best with a water extraction, like a tea or decoction. In a tincture of alcohol, we draw out different chemical components, vinegar attracts the nutrients, and animal or vegetable glycerin is less potent and gentler for older and younger folk. We can infuse herbs in vegetable oils, then apply the oil on the skin for wounds, skin care, or in massage. We are looking for the most favorable process to release the healing constituents without shattering the medicinal healing properties.

PLANT TEAS

Herbal teas are water infusions made from the delicate parts of the plants, like the flower, leaf, and crushed seed.

1 tablespoon dried herb
1 cup (240 ml) hot water

Place the herbal material in a teacup with the water and let steep for 5 to 30 minutes, or longer for a stronger tea. For a teapot portion, add more herbal material, about 4 to 6 tablespoons, and adjust the water accordingly.

SOLAR AND LUNAR INFUSIONS

Solar and lunar infusions are ancient ways of preparing medicine where we enlist the energy of the sun or moon to gently extract or release the herbal healing properties. Place fresh or dried herbal parts in a glass jar, cover with water, and put it in direct sun for several hours or in the moonlight overnight.

DECOCTIONS

Decoctions are water infusions simmered over long periods with dense herbal material like roots, larger seeds, and bark. Because this herbal material is denser and harder in structure, they need more time to release and infuse the chemical compounds into the liquid.

Handful of dried dense plant material
1 to 2 quarts (1 to 2 L) water

Add your herbal material and water to a pot and let simmer for 5 to 30 minutes, then cover with a lid. Notice the color of your decoction and the fragrance that arises. I like an overnight decoction, where you pour boiling water over the plant material, cover with a lid, and let it steep until the following morning. This process allows for more minerals to be released. Gently warm up should you prefer a hot tea to drink.

TINCTURES

A tincture is a more concentrated infusion using alcohol or animal/vegetable glycerin as a base. The question is: Is it best to use dry or fresh herbal material? Some research suggests that dried herbs make a more stable extract and have a longer shelf life. Tinctures made from fresh herb material are less stable and generally weaker in terms of expression of the dissolved phytochemicals, as the plant materials still contain water. When tinctures are made with dried herbs, the alcohol penetrates the cells and it is a more efficient extraction of the phyto-active properties. All that being said, preference is based on individual herbs. The 1:2 ratio of herb material to alcohol or glycerin is a standard formula, and when dividing deeper into tinctures, there are a multitude of specific ratios for various herbs. Tinctures can last up to 10 years.

1:2 ratio of plant material to alcohol or glycerin

Mix medicines in a glass jar and leave to infuse for 4 weeks in a dark cupboard. Label with the name and the date and moon phase of when you collected. Strain out the herbal material and bottle as desired. For quick absorption, use drops under your tongue. Should this be too strong, add to juice or a hot tea as the hot water will help evaporate the alcohol, or consider rubbing a few drops on the bottom of your feet and massaging it in.

HYDROSOLS

Place a rock or metal pedestal with an empty metal bowl on top into a large soup pot. Fill the soup pot with the herb material and water until it surrounds the pedestal and empty bowl. Place the lid on top of the pot upside down and fill it with ice cubes. Bring the water to a simmer and watch closely so as not to burn. As the steam rises, it will hit the cool lid and the condensed steam will drip into the metal bowl. Depending on the density of the herb, it can take 30 minutes to 1 hour or longer to distill the aerosols. Strain and bottle, or pour into spray bottles. Label and store in your fridge.

VINEGAR TINCTURES

Vinegar infusions extract minerals and vitamins, such as calcium, iron, potassium, and vitamin C, from the herb material. Use any type of vinegar except white vinegar, which is mostly made with bioengineered corn. I prefer apple cider vinegar for its flavor.

1:2 ratio of dried herb material to vinegar of choice

Place the herb material in a glass jar and cover with vinegar, ensuring the liquid does not touch the lid. Shake daily and steep for 4 weeks. Strain, bottle, and label.

NOTE: Dried herbs are best to avoid adding water content into the vinegar, which makes for a less stable product.

SYRUPS

Syrups are a great choice for children because the base to carry the medicine is honey, maple syrup, sugar, or vegetable glycerin. Honey-based medicines are not suitable for kids under two years old.

NOTE: A basic ratio recipe is 2 parts herbal materials to 1 part honey or sugar, for example, 2 cups (480 ml) herbal materials to 1 cup (240 ml) sweetener. Other recipes may suggest a 1:1 ratio of herbal materials to sweetener. You may find this too sweet. Experiment with the recipe to find what works best. Notice if the aromatics are strong in their aroma then use ⅓ cup (80 ml). For example with rosemary or thyme. For strong flavors like lavender use only 2 to 3 tablespoons (30 to 45 ml). Rose petals up to 2 cups (480 ml). To flavor with lemon, add 1 cup (240 ml) juice and 1 tablespoon (15 ml) lemon zest.

½ cup (120 ml) to 1 cup (240 ml) herbal material. Amount depends upon density of the plant.
2 cups (240 ml) water
¼ cup (60 ml) to ½ cup (120 ml) sweetener (honey, maple syrup, sugar, or glycerin)
Optional 1 tablespoon (15 ml) alcohol such as brandy

Add the herb material and water to a saucepan and simmer over low heat. Reduce the liquid by half. Strain and pour the liquid back into the pot. Add the sweetener and gently heat until blended together. Remove from the heat, let cool, add the brandy, and bottle. The syrup will keep for several weeks and longer when stored in the fridge.

GUMMIES

Gummies are easy to make using homemade syrup (recipe above) as a base.

3 to 5 tablespoons dried herbal material or dried vitamin powder
3 tablespoons gelatin
½ cup (120 ml) fruit juice of choice, at room temperature
½ cup (120 ml) homemade syrup

Place the dried herb material in a bowl and put aside. In a separate bowl, add the gelatin and fruit juice. Stir and let sit for a few minutes until dissolved. In a saucepan, warm up the homemade syrup but don't boil. Add the dissolved gelatin and fruit juice mixture to the warmed syrup and whisk quickly. Remove from the heat and mix in the dry ingredients. Gently pour into molds or on parchment paper and put in the freezer for an hour until it sets. Pop out the gummies from the molds or cut the set mixture into bite-size pieces; store in an airtight container for up to 2 weeks in the fridge. Take 1 to 3 gummies per day, less for children.

NOTE: If there is a lot of vitamin C powder in your gummies, you may notice your stool is loose.

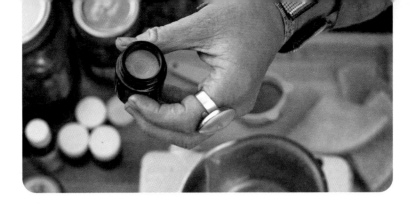

INFUSED OILS

Infused oils are a soothing way to administer plants' healing medicine through the skin. Infused oils are the base for making facial oils, salves, ointments, massage oils, and creams. Choose which base you like most: Olive oil, coconut oil, sunflower oil, jojoba oil, almond oil, avocado oil, etc.

1:2 ratio of dried herb material to oil of your choice

Finely chop the herb material or add to a blender and blend thoroughly, and then pour into a clean jar and cover with oil. Shake the jar daily, making sure no herb material is poking outside the mixture to avoid the infusion going moldy. Keep in a dark area away from sunlight. Allow 4 to 6 weeks for the medicine to extract into the oil. Strain into a clean jar or bottle and label.

SALVES, OINTMENTS, AND LIP BALMS

Salves, ointments, and lip balms are made from infused oils (recipe above). Salves are slightly firmer than an ointment, and lip balms will be even firmer than a salve.

1:5 ratio of beeswax to infused oil or 3 1/2 tablespoons (50 ml) beeswax
to 1 cup (240 ml) oil, at room temperature

Break the beeswax into similar sizes so it melts easily and consistently. Add the beeswax to a double boiler and let it melt. Then add the infused oil and stir. When adding the oil, it will change the temperature of the melted beeswax and coagulate, making it look like egg soup. Stir occasionally until the wax is fully melted. With a spoon, scoop out a little and let cool. This will let you know if you need to adjust the firmness. Add drops of essential oil if you prefer extra scent with added healing properties. Once it has reached your desired consistency, pour into clean containers and let cool. Label and share the gifts. Typically the product will last one year.

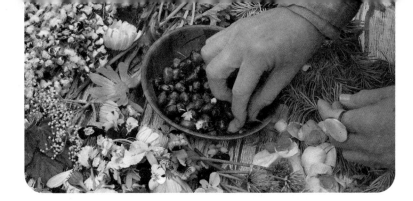

LINIMENTS

Liniments are made the same way as alcohol-based tinctures except the menstruum (solvent) is rubbing alcohol or witch hazel extract. Use only externally for sore muscles or as a disinfectant.

1:2 ratio of herb material to rubbing alcohol or witch hazel extract

Steep the plant material in the rubbing alcohol for 4 weeks, then strain into a clean bottle and label appropriately.

POULTICES

A poultice is a paste of heated pulverized or chopped herbs. Apply either directly to the skin or wrap up in a clean cloth and then apply to the body. The heat increases blood flow to the area, heating the properties of the herb for better absorption. Poultices can be made with clay, mud, or various vegetables like onions or potatoes.

INCENSE

Incense cones are a great gift to mold with our hands and give to our loved ones. Collect fragrant plant materials, aromatic fallen tree branches, rose petals, old spices, powdered orange or lemon peels, and marshmallow root; the root is the binder or glue in this recipe. You can also grow your own marshmallow root, then dry it and grind it into powder. You will need a coffee grinder for this, preferably one only used for herbs and spices.

1 tablespoon dried plant material, 1 teaspoon marshmallow root
1 teaspoon water, or more as needed

Using your hands, combine the plant material and marshmallow root in a bowl. Add the water and mix well. Add more water as needed. Mold into a conical shape, like a Christmas tree with a pointy tip. Let dry on the countertop for 5 days or place in the oven overnight with the oven light on. NOTE: Burn responsibly. Say your prayers and know that you are disinfecting your space with aromatics to keep yourself and your loved ones healthy.

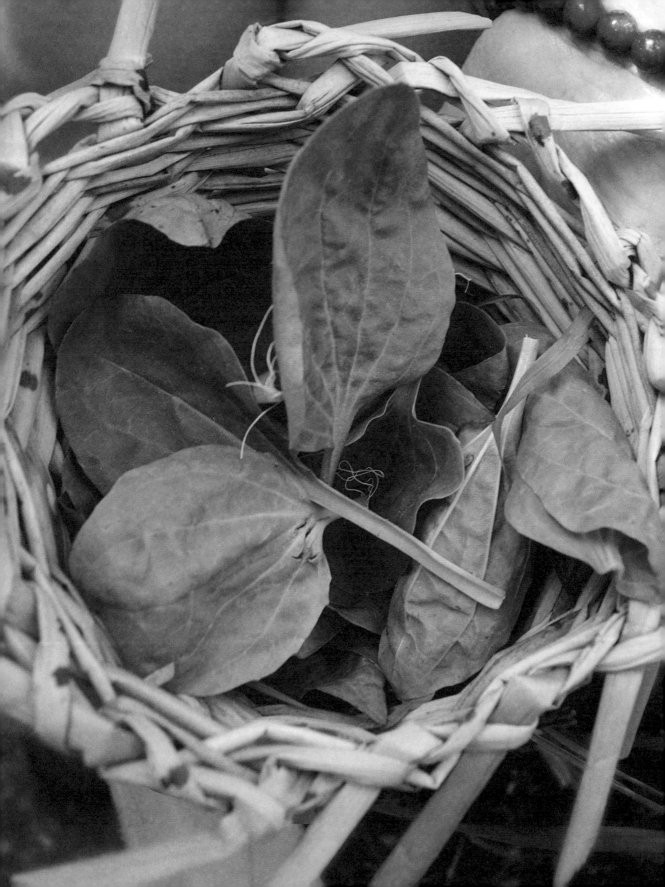

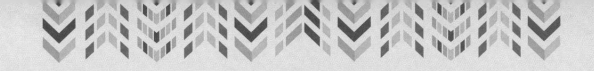

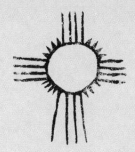

Reflections
of Deep Reverence

Ablution (noun), the act of washing oneself. Washing, cleansing, a ceremonial act of washing parts of the body or a scared vessel.

Heal yourself with the light of the sun and the rays of the moon.
With the sound of the river and the waterfall.
With the swaying of the sea and the fluttering of birds.
Heal yourself with mint, neem, and eucalyptus.
Sweeten with lavender, rosemary, and chamomile.
Hug yourself with the cocoa bean and a touch of cinnamon.
Put love in your tea instead of sugar and drink it looking at the stars.
Heal yourself with the kisses that the wind gives to you and the hugs of the rain.
Stand strong with your bare feet on the ground and with everything that comes from it.
Get smarter every day by listening to your intuition and
looking at the world with the eye of your forehead.
Jump, dance, sing, so that you live happier.
Heal yourself with beautiful love, and always remember,
you are the medicine.

by Maria Sabina Magdalena Garcia (1894–1985),
a *sabia* (wise woman), shaman (Mazatec spiritual healer),
and poet from Oaxaca, Mexico

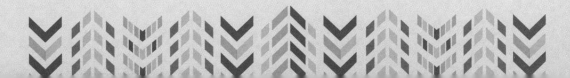

Glossary ACTIONS OF PLANT USE

Our botanical herbs can be classified as having a rapport, an affinity, for certain organ systems or are suited for a specific quality. Here is a small sampling of "actions" to start you on the journey with a few examples.

Alterative Cleanses the blood to restore the proper function of the body and increases health and vitality. Examples: cleavers, echinacea, stinging nettles, red clover, yellow dock.

Analgesic Reduces pain and can be applied externally or taken internally. Examples: willow bark, valerian, St. John's wort.

Anthelmintic Expels worms from the digestive tract. Examples: garlic, aloe vera.

Antibilious Helps remove excessive bile, such as with jaundice. Examples: dandelion, mugwort, vervain.

Anti-catarrhal Helps break up and remove excess mucus. Examples: peppermint, yarrow, echinacea, garlic, mullein.

Antiemetic Relieves nausea or vomiting. Examples: raspberry leaf, lavender, meadowsweet, fennel, ginger.

Anti-inflammatory Reduces inflammation externally and/or internally. Examples: willow, chamomile, fireweed, calendula, St. John's wort, witch hazel.

Antilithic Prevents the formation and aids in dissolving of stones and gravel in the urinary system. Examples: corn silk, parsley, bearberry, hydrangea.

Antimicrobial Destroys or resists pathogenic microorganisms. Examples: bearberry, juniper, peppermint, calendula, echinacea, clove, sage, lavender.

Antispasmodic Eases spasms or cramps. Examples: chamomile, black cohosh, thyme, valerian, vervain, cramp bark.

Aromatic Has a strong scent to help stimulate digestion. Examples: chamomile, fennel, dill, ginger, rosemary, cardamom.

Astringent Contracts tissue by triggering proteins, reducing secretions, and discharging tannins. Examples: bearberry, plantain, raspberry leaf, rosemary, slippery elm, St. John's wort, yarrow.

Bitters Stimulates the digestion system, starting with saliva. Examples: yarrow, chamomile, dandelion leaf, gentian.

Cardiac Works on the heart. Examples: hawthorn, motherwort.

Carminative Relaxes the stomach, supporting digestion and relieving bloating and gas. Examples: fennel, juniper berry, chamomile, cinnamon, ginger, peppermint, thyme, valerian.

Cholagogue Stimulates the gallbladder for the secretion of bile and a laxative effect. Examples: dandelion root, barberry, gentian, wild yam.

Demulcent Soothes and protects irritated or inflamed internal tissue. Examples: licorice, corn silk, comfrey, flax seed, slippery elm, parsley, lungwort.

Diaphoretic Aids the skin to eliminate toxins by promoting perspiration. Examples: ginger, thyme, yarrow, peppermint, cayenne, fennel, prickly ash.

Diuretic Stimulates kidney function by increasing the elimination of urine. Examples: borage, burdock, celery seed, cleavers, corn silk, dandelion, hawthorn berries, stinging nettle, yarrow.

Emetic Causes vomiting at higher dosages. Example: elderflower.

Emmenagogue Stimulates and balances menstrual flow. Examples: ginger, raspberry leaf, rosemary, chastetree, cramp bark, blue cohosh, mugwort, raspberry leaf, yarrow.

Emollient Applied to the skin to soften, soothe, and protect. Examples: borage, chickweed, comfrey, marshmallow, mullein, plantain.

Expectorant Works with the respiratory system to support in the removal of excess mucus. Examples: comfrey, elderflower, garlic, lobelia, licorice, wild cherry bark.

Febrifuge Helps the body lower the temperature of a fever. Examples: blessed thistle, borage, cayenne, elderflower, peppermint, raspberry leaf, thyme.

Galactagogue Promotes and increases breast milk flow. Examples: aniseed, blessed thistle, fennel, borage.

Hepatic Tones and strengthens the liver and increases the flow of bile. Examples: aloe vera, cleavers, dandelion, fennel, goldenseal, motherwort, yarrow, yellow dock.

Hypnotic Helps induce sleep. Examples: chamomile, hops, passionflower, skullcap, valerian.

Laxative Promotes the evacuation of the bowels. Examples: burdock, cascara sagrada, dandelion, flax seed, senna, yellow dock.

Nervine Tones and strengthens the nervous system, either stimulating or relaxing. Examples: black cohosh, chamomile, damiana, ginseng, hops, lavender, lemon balm, oatstraw, peppermint, red clover, rosemary.

Oxytocic Stimulates contractions of the uterus and can be helpful with childbirth. Examples: blue cohosh, squaw vine, goldenseal.

Pectoral Has general strengthening and healing effects on the respiratory system. Examples: comfrey, garlic, elderflower, Irish moss, licorice, lungwort, mullein, marshmallow.

Rubefacient Causes local reddening of the skin through activating blood circulation, reaching deeper layers in the skin. Can help with internal pain. Examples: mustard, cayenne, stinging nettles, horseradish, ginger.

Sedative Calms the nervous system and reduces tension. Examples: blue cohosh, chamomile, hops, passionflower, St. John's wort, red clover, skullcap.

Stimulant Enlivens the physiological functions of the whole body. Examples: angelica, juniper berry, caraway, rosemary, sage, yarrow, cinnamon, pennyroyal.

Styptic Reduces or stops external bleeding through their astringent nature. Examples: bearberry, eyebright, goldenrod, lungwort, usnea, plantain, rhubarb root, yarrow.

Tonic Strengthens and tones a targeted organ or the whole body. Examples: aniseed, black cohosh, burdock, cleavers, yellow dock, yarrow, dandelion, hawthorn, goldenseal, ginseng, unicorn root, sarsaparilla, mugwort, oatstraw, wood betony, gravel root, stinging nettles, parsley, echinacea, coltsfoot.

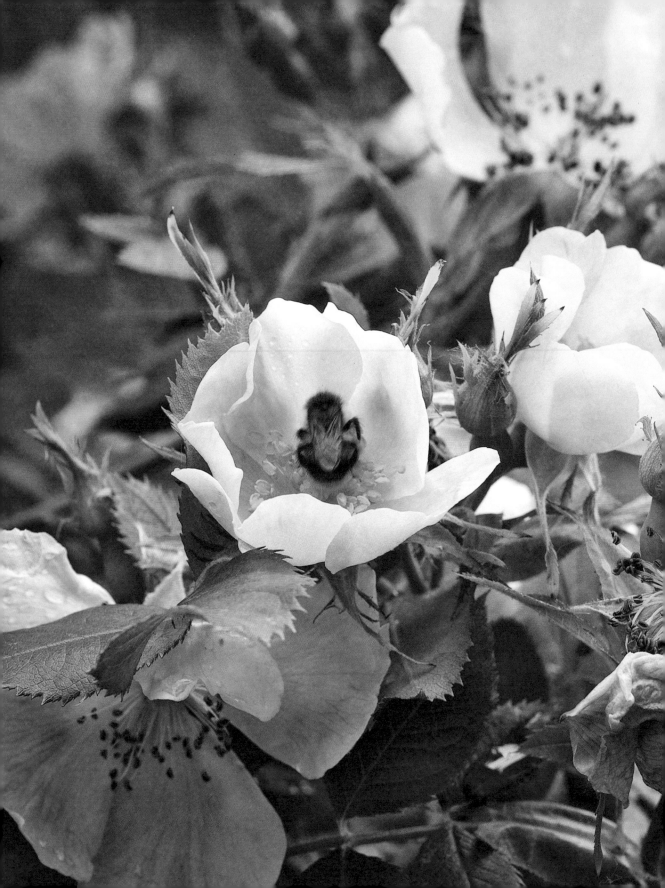

Acknowledgments

We have our instructions, medicines to help us, and references like *Held by the Land*; *Gathering Moss*; *We Are the ARK: Returning Our Gardens to Their True Nature Through Acts of Restorative Kindness*; *Plants Have So Much to Give Us, All We Have to Do Is Ask*.

I am humbled, grateful, and blessed for the forces that have shaped and guided my spirit to this moment. My ancestors from both sides of the ocean. My mother, Esther, and my father, Bert. My spiritual parents of the mountains and waters of the land I was born on. My next-door neighbor, Mrs. Bruun, who started me on the path, just by introducing me to the Rooted Nations, my plant Elders. My first herb teacher, Don Ollsin, my "herby sisters," and all the other sisters I met along the way, sharing these teachings and friendship.

Hands up to Della (Rice) Sylvester, *Huyamise*, from the Cowichan People who helped answered my question, "Should I teach children?" This book is for our children's children. To *Ta7taliya* Michelle Nahanee from the Squamish Nation, who welcomed me with kindness and is a brilliant educator on decolonizing practices. To my dear "herb sister," Jeri Sparrow from the Musqueam Nation, with whom I can sit, drink tea, and swap stories. And to my new relations with the Tsleil-Waututh Nation.

I hold my hands up for my spirit guides and the falcon who appeared yesterday, who brings vision, who can look beyond the immediate horizon toward a future filled with possibilities. To focus, commit, overcome obstacles, and remain centered. A messenger who encourages us to seize opportunities with boldness, respond when the time is right, and move toward the future with determination and speed.

To Stephanie Rose, a dear sister and editor, for her prayers, answered, to see me write this book, and Jessica Walliser, my acquiring editor, who took a risk and jumped in.

To my second mom and friend, Margaret Rose, who listens so well, and to her son, Steven Charles, who partnered with me to birth two beautiful, bright daughters into the world.

To the Rooted Nations, who have loved me along the way to be of service to all that exists, the bridge to my human ancestors. I have learned a lot about myself, that I can be slow like a turtle, reflected in my dear sister from the Caribbean Sea. Thank you to my own present health challenges that keep me humble and committed to my own health.

LM, LJ, ER, VJ, this book is for you. I love you all to the moon and back.

All our Relations.
LoriAnn Bird

P.S. Any one of my Indigenous Relatives from Turtle Island who would like a copy of *Revered Roots*, please get in touch with me and I will send a copy to your Nation or Tribe.
In Ojibwe, we say, *Chi miigwech* (big thank you).
In Kichwa, we say, *Ashka pakrachu* (universal love).
In Shuar, we say, *Yuminsajme.* (There are no equivalent English words to express our gratitude for life.)

References

David Abram. 1996. *The Spell of the Sensuous: Perception and Language in a More-Than-Human World*. New York: Pantheon Books.

Doug Anderson, Julie Comay, and Lorriane Chiarotto. 2017. *Natural Curiosity: The Importance of Indigenous Perspectives in Children's Environmental Inquiry*. Toronto: The Laboratory School at the Dr. Eric Jackman Institute of Child Study.

Thomas Bartram. 1995. *Bartram's Encyclopedia of Herbal Medicine: The Definitive Guide to the Herbal Treatment of Diseases*. London: Robinson Publishing Ltd.

Christi Belcourt. 2007. *Medicines to Help Us: Traditional Métis Plant Use*. Contributions by Elders Rose Richardson and Olive Whitford. Saskatoon, Canada: The Gabriel Dumont Institute of Native Studies and Applied Research.

Thomas Berry. 1988. *The Dream of the Earth. Sierra Club Nature and Natural Philosophy Library*. San Francisco: Sierra Club Books.

Katrina Blair. 2014. *The Wild Wisdom of Weeds: 13 Essential Plants for Human Survival*. White River Junction, VT: Chelsea Green Publishing.

Michael J. Caduto and Joseph Bruchac. 1996. *Native American Gardening: Stories, Projects, and Recipes for Families*. Golden, CO: Fulcrum Publishing.

Luschiim Arvid Charlie and Nancy J. Turner. 2021. *Luschiim's Plants: Traditional Indigenous Foods, Materials, and Medicines*. Madeira Park, BC, Canada: Harbour Publishing.

Joe Dispenza. 2017. *Becoming Supernatural: How Common People Are Doing the Uncommon*. Carlsbad, CA: Hay House.

Rosalee De La Foret and Emily Han. 2020. *Wild Remedies: How to Forage Healing Foods and Craft Your Own Herbal Medicine*. Carlsbad, CA: Hay House.

Mary Siisip Geniusz. 2015. *Plants Have So Much to Give Us, All We Have to Do Is Ask: Anishinaabe Botanical Teachings*. Minneapolis, MN: University of Minnesota Press.

Chief Dan George. 1989. *My Heart Soars*. Surrey, Canada: Hancock House Publishers.

Euell Gibbons. 1962. *Stalking the Wild Asparagus: Field Guide Edition*. New York: David McKay Company Inc.

Beverly Gray. 2011. *The Boreal Herbal: Wild Food and Medicine Plants of the North*. Whitehorse, Yukon, Canada: Aroma Borealis Press.

GRuB and Northwest Indian Treatment Center. 2020. *Plant Teachings for Growing Social-Emotional Skills: Cultivating Resiliency and Wellbeing with Northwest Plants*. Seattle, WA: GRuB 2020, Creative Commons.

David R. Hawkins. 1995. *Power vs. Force: The Hidden Determinants of Human Behavior*. Carlsbad, CA: Hay House.

David Hoffmann. 2003. *Medical Herbalism: The Science and Practice of Herbal Medicine*. Rochester, VT: Healing Arts Press.

Alma R. Hutchens. 1974. *Indian Herbalogy of North America: The Definitive Guide to Native Medicinal Plants and Their Uses*. Boston: Shambhala Publications, Inc.

Leigh Joseph. 2023. *Held by the Land: A Guide to Indigenous Plants for Wellness*. New York: Quarto Publishing Group.

Robin Wall Kimmerer. 2013. *Braiding Sweetgrass: Indigenous Wisdom, Scientific Knowledge, and the Teachings of Plants*. Minneapolis: Milkweed Editions.

Wab Kinew. 2015. *The Reason You Walk*. Toronto: Penguin.

La Societe Historique de Saint-Boniface 2000. *Ancestors of Lori Snyder (nee Biglow)*.

Joseph Marshall III. 2012. *The Lakota Way of Strength and Courage: Lessons in Resilience from the Bow and Arrow.* Boulder, CO: Sounds True.

Daniel E. Moerman. 1998. *Native American Ethnobotany*. Portland, OR: Timber Press.

Michael Moore. 1993. *Medicinal Plants of the Pacific West*. Santa Fe: Museum of New Mexico Press.

The Ojibwe People's Dictionary. https://ojibwe.lib.umn.edu.

Don Ollsin. 2000. *Pathways to Healing: A Guide to Herbs, Ayurveda, Dreambody, and Shamanism*. Toronto: Frog Books.

Joseph Pitawanakwat. YouTube. Creatorsgardenmarket.ca.

Jim Pojar and Andy MacKinnon. 1994. *Plants of Coastal British Columbia, Including Washington, Oregon, and Alaska*. Vancouver: Lone Pine Publishing.

Mary Reynolds. 2022. *We Are the Ark: Returning Our Gardens to Their True Nature with Acts of Restorative Kindness*. Portland, OR: Timber Press.

Stephanie Rose. 2020. *Garden Alchemy: 80 Recipes and Concoctions for Organic Fertilizers, Plant Elixirs, Potting Mixes, Pest Deterrents, and More*. New York: Quarto Group.

Enrique Salmon. 2020. *IWIGARA: The Kinship of Plant and People: American Indian Ethnobotanical Traditions and Science*. Portland, OR: Timber Press.

Janice J. Schofield. 1996. *Discovering Wild Plants: Alaska, Western Canada, The Northwest*. Portland, OR: Graphic Arts Center Publishing.

Susanne Simard. 2021. *Finding the Mother Tree: Discovering the Wisdom of the Forest*. Toronto: Penguin Random House.

Adam F. Szczawinski and Nancy J. Turner. 1978. *Edible Garden Weeds of Canada*. Ottawa: National Museum of Canada.

Doug Tallamy. https://homegrownnationalpark.org.

Susun S. Weed. 2002. *New Menopausal Years: The Wise Woman Way: Alternative Approaches for Women 30–90.* Woodstock, NY: Ash Tree Publishing.

Matthew Wood. 1997. *The Book of Herbal Wisdom: Using Plants as Medicines*. Berkeley, CA: North Atlantic Books.

George Woodcock. 1975. *Gabriel Dumont: The Métis Chief and His Lost World*. Edmonton, Canada: Hurtig Publishers.

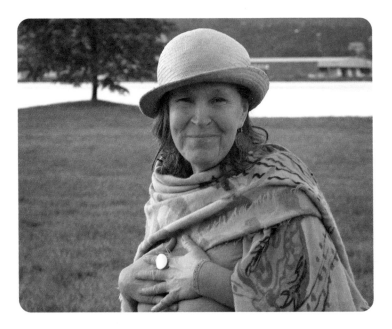

About the Author

LoriAnn Bird is a mother of two daughters and a storyteller who educates about wild, native, and medicinal plants. Her heritage is a blend of many cultures from Turtle Island and Europe that weave her unique heritage. She loves exploring the connection between people and our More-Than-Human-Kin, the plants that offer many teachings. Such plants grow in everyday spaces, opening our perspective to our immediate surroundings and engaging in a new relationship as we see the wealth of untapped life-giving, ecological gifts that are given.

LoriAnn leads folks of diverse backgrounds in reconnecting to Mother Earth's wisdom in various workshops that she offers. LoriAnn's vision is to continually co-create dialogues, to remediate and reconcile with all of our relatives. By sharing and growing "wild spaces," communities can access our true local foods and medicines, which support collective, resilient, and deep, restorative healing. She says, "I pray that we plant tree nurseries under the Grandmother Trees, that we collaborate with our More-Than-Human-Kin, co-creating harvesting corridors down back alleys, along edges of parks, in schoolyards, and in other open spaces."

Reach out for information on projects in the Ecuadorian rainforest. Visit LoriAnn @ https://loriannbird.ca

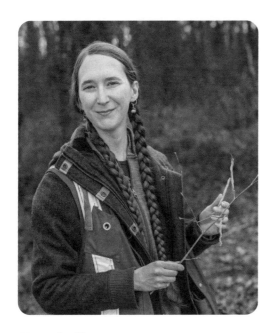

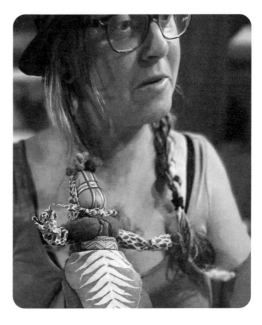

About the Illustrator

Julia Alards-Tomalin is an instructor in the Renewable Resources department at the British Columbia Institute of Technology (BCIT), in Burnaby, Canada. She is currently the Program Head for the Forest and Natural Areas Management program. She studied Forestry and Ecological Restoration at BCIT and completed a Master of Education at Simon Fraser University. Her background is diverse, including horticulture, arboriculture, urban forestry and ecological restoration, but is united by a common theme of plants. Her interest in plants has been a life-long endeavour and has inspired her to co-create a Youtube Channel: Interviews with Plants, and a winter plant identification textbook: Buds, Branches and Bark: A Guide to Winter ID in the Pacific Northwest. Learn more at:

www.bcit.ca/open/faculty-in-the-open/julia-alards-tomalin/

About the Photographer

Belinda is a deep nature connection mentor for children and adults in Vancouver and beyond, a photographer, and a storyteller who lives and breathes the art and magic of weaving with image and word.

She dwells at the intersections of story, nature connection, art, and cultural repair through documentation, writing, poetry, workshop, and ritual. Belinda came to this work through the struggles of raising a child through divorce and without an extended village. Along the way, she has carried two enduring questions: What is it that connects us deeply to life? Can disconnection be repaired? She has found that her wild kin offer immeasurable support through earth arts, plant medicine, and more. Belinda believes "The stories we tell are the stories we live by."

Belinda's desire is to weave a basket of belonging through visual and oral storytelling, mentoring, inner tracking, and grief tending among others. If you'd like to contact Belinda about photography or her other projects, you can find her on Instagram and Facebook @applestarphoto @theTwiningTrail @apple_star_learning.

Index

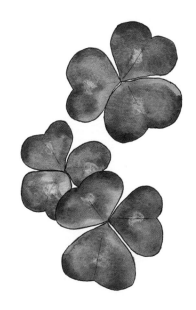

motherwort, 126
mouthwash, 75, 92, 99, 141, 144
mucus, 44, 63, 121, 168, 178
mullein, 123–125
mycorrhizal network, 16–17

N

natural cycles, 12, 36–37
natural laws, 15, 16–17
nausea, 68, 73, 97, 104, 117, 210
Nepeta cataria, 94–95
nephritis, 136
nervine, 89, 126
nervous system, 50, 60, 83, 85,
    87, 98, 118, 134, 150, 162
nettle, purple dead, 70–71
neurotoxins, 29
Nicotiana genus, 30–31
nicotine, 30–31
night sweats, 83
nodding onion, 66–67
nonnative plants, 19
nosebleeds, 72, 91

O

oatstraw, 84–85
ointments, 224
Ollsin, Don, 25
Oregon grape, 127–129
ovarian cancer, 64
Oxalis acetosella, 68–69
Oxalis oregana, 68–69
oxeye daisy, 82–83

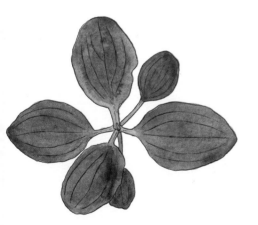

P

pain relief, 31, 102, 103, 172, 189,
    198, 204, 212
Panax quinquefolius, 159
paper birch, 64–65
partridgeberry, 150–151
Passiflora incarnata, 112–113
passionflower, 112–113
pearly everlasting, 140–141
peppermint, 96–97
phenolic, 200
phlegm, 146, 187, 204
phytol, 33
pine, 46–47
pine pollen, 56–57
pink eye, 108
Pinus genus, 56–57
Pitawanakwat, Joseph, 34
Plantago lanceolata, 41
Plantago major, 41
plantain, 41
plants
    relationship with, 27, 37
    vital spirit of, 27
PMS (premenstrual syndrome),
    106, 110, 126
Podophyllum peltatum, 196–197
poison hemlock, 73, 185
poison sumac, 157
Populus genus, 198–199
Portulaca oleracea, 78–79
poultices, 225
prickly ash, 160–161
propolis, 170–171
prostate, 48, 57, 80, 110, 122,
    132, 176, 194
prostatitis, 50
Prunus genus, 86–88
psoriasis, 45, 50, 145, 194
psychiatric disorders, 190
purple dead nettle, 70–71
purslane, 78–79

Q

Q'ero People, 13

R

rashes, 64, 72, 108, 148, 156, 174,
    198
raspberry leaf, red, 52–53
reciprocity, 21, 27

red osier dogwood, 216–217
red raspberry leaf, 52–53
Red River Métis People, 12
relationships, 19
reproductive health, 68, 150, 182.
    See also menstruation
reptiles, 22
respect, 16–17
responsibility, 15
reverence, 22–23
Rhamnus purshiana, 209
rheumatism, 75, 100, 160, 172,
    174, 182, 194, 197, 210
Rhus glabra, 156–157
Rooted Nations, 12, 13, 19, 25,
    27, 125
rosacea, 42
Rosa genus, 192–193
rose, 192–193
rosemary, 100–101
Rosmarinus officinalis, 100–101
Rubus idaeus, 52–53
Rubus species, 142–143
Rudbeckia hirta, 152–153
Rumex acetosella, 68–69
Rumex crispus, 44–45

S

sage, 28–29
Sagittaria latifolia, 154–155
Salix species, 103–105
Salmon, Enrique, 32
salves, 224
Salvia apiana, 28–29
Salvia officinalis, 98–99
Sambucus genus, 114–115
saskatoon berry, 138–139
scarlet pimpernel, 43
scars, 58, 108, 135
sciatica pain, 89, 135, 189, 202
scurvy, 46, 68, 180
seasonal affect disorder (SAD), 134
sedatives, 54, 87, 88, 89, 98, 121,
    140
self, responsibility to, 15
serotonin, 36
shingles, 89, 135
Silybum marianum, 122
Simard, Suzanne, 16
skin conditions, 42, 64, 75, 104,
    108, 127, 143, 144–145, 148,
    152, 160, 172, 174, 176, 194,
    198, 202, 210, 214

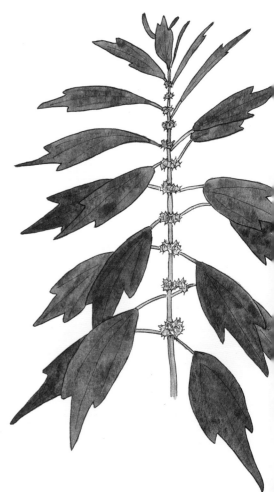